ADVANCE PRAISE

"[This book is] packed full of useful information patients can put to good use immediately to help them heal faster and get back to the things they enjoy. Using easy-to-understand examples, this book helps guide patients through the stressful pre-surgical period to become stronger and healthier for whatever lies ahead. This book is a must for anyone preparing for surgery or other major medical treatment. Even a short time of preparing your body with the right nutrition, exercise, and mental conditioning can make a big difference in recovery."
—KAREN BARR, DO, SOLID ORGAN TRANSPLANT PREHABILITATION SPECIALIST, UNIVERSITY OF PITTSBURGH MEDICAL CENTER

"As a physical therapist, I have spent years trying to educate my patients so they can be more in charge of their health. With this book, Dr. Watson takes that concept and lays out a framework for those coming to terms with a life-changing diagnosis or while preparing for an elective procedure. Now, these patients have the resources needed to navigate the next step in their journey, optimized for the best possible outcome."
—LAUREN GRIEDER, PT, DPT, OCS, SCS

"Dr. Watson absolutely delivers! As a rehabilitation physician, Dr. Watson is an expert in all phases of the rehabilitation process. In this exciting read, rich with practical information and tips, he covers the importance of the "pre-habilitation" process. Dr. Watson shares his vast knowledge to anticipate and address key factors to optimize functional performance and outcomes from surgery and illness. In health, prevention is everything. Get the insight you need to thrive in Healing in Advance by Alexander Watson, MD."

—JUSTIN BERTHOLD, DO, REHABILITATION PHYSICIANS OF PITTSBURGH

HEALING IN ADVANCE

HEALING IN *ADVANCE*

Your *P*rehabilitation Handbook

ALEXANDER WATSON, MD

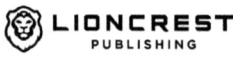

COPYRIGHT © 2025 ALEXANDER WATSON
All rights reserved.

HEALING IN ADVANCE
Your Prehabilitation Handbook

FIRST EDITION

ISBN 978-1-5445-4666-7 Hardcover
      978-1-5445-4665-0 Paperback
      978-1-5445-4667-4 Ebook

To Wes. Right now, you're too young to pronounce "prehabilitation," let alone understand why, after writing an entire book, this dedication is the only place I mention dinosaurs. Work hard at something you love, my little Wesleysaurus, and no matter what I'll be proud of you.

CONTENTS

FOREWORD 11
INTRODUCTION 15

PART I
1. THE RECIPE FOR PREHABILITATION SUCCESS .. 27
2. DIAGNOSTICS AND MEETING YOUR MEDS 75

PART II
3. ORTHOPEDIC PREHABILITATION 135
4. CANCER TREATMENT PREHABILITATION 155
5. BARIATRIC SURGERY PREHABILITATION 181
6. AMPUTEE PREHABILITATION 207
7. TRANSPLANT PREHABILITATION 229
8. FERTILITY, GYNECOLOGIC SURGERY, AND UROLOGIC SURGERY PREHABILITATION 249
9. OUR MISSION TO PUT HEALING FIRST 267

ACKNOWLEDGMENTS 271
ABOUT THE AUTHOR 273

FOREWORD

—YEHUDA "YUDI" KERBEL, MD
FELLOWSHIP-TRAINED
ORTHOPEDIC SURGEON

SOME OF MY SICKEST PATIENTS ARE STUCK IN A CRUEL CATCH-22. They're too sick for surgery, yet their bad hips or knees stop them from exercising. On top of that, many need to lose weight, but because of diseases like diabetes, they eat around the clock or else their insulin makes their blood sugar fall too low. It's a vicious cycle that can feel impossible to break. Their health is trapped in a web of medical conditions, each worsening the others, and their spirits are often weighed down by the frustration and helplessness that come from this unending loop. For these patients, the path to recovery can seem like an impassable mountain.

This is where the elegance of Dr. Watson's approach comes into play. Dr. Watson lays out a roadmap that is easy to remember and even easier to follow. Everyone has their own unique journey, which means no single plan can work for all patients.

Conveniently, this book includes several ways to attack each of the dozens of potential roadblocks and detours along anyone's prehabilitation journey. It's not a one-size-fits-all solution; instead, it's a dynamic and adaptable guide that respects the individuality of each patient and their specific circumstances.

In the years I have spent as an orthopedic surgeon, I have learned that the period leading up to surgery can be as crucial as the surgery itself; in some cases, poor health can derail surgical plans completely. The concept of prehabilitation—or prehab—has transformed the way I approach patient care for patients with complex medical needs. Prehab is about preparing the body in the best possible way for the stresses of surgery. It's about building strength, improving nutrition, and optimizing overall health to ensure that patients are not only ready for surgery but also set up for the best possible recovery. And Dr. Watson's book is a master class in this essential process.

The uniqueness of each patient's journey cannot be overstated. Some patients come to me with severe joint pain that has kept them nearly immobile for months or even years. Others struggle with obesity, a condition that complicates their health in myriad ways and adds significant risk to any surgical procedure. Still others are battling chronic illnesses like diabetes that require careful management of their diet and medications. Each of these factors presents a unique challenge that must be addressed through a tailored prehab plan, anticipating how each could produce specific complications during and after surgery.

This book is a treasure trove of strategies and insights, meticulously designed to help patients overcome these obstacles. For instance, patients with severe joint pain are given gentle, low-impact exercises that help them build strength. These are paired with pain management strategies that are more than just opioids and ibuprofen. Those struggling with weight issues will find nutritional nuggets that are both practical and sustainable, helping them lose weight without feeling overly deprived. Diabetic patients are guided through specific dietary adjustments and exercise routines that help manage their blood sugar levels effectively.

I've noticed that the patients who do best after surgery are the ones who, despite hectic jobs and busy families, find a little time every day to prioritize their health. These are the patients who follow a prehabilitation plan and go into surgery feeling even better than they did at their initial surgical consultation. This book helps focus that preparation, maximizing benefits with the least required time and no wasted effort. It's about smart, targeted interventions that yield significant results, enabling patients to approach their surgeries with confidence and resilience.

One of the most rewarding aspects of my practice is witnessing the transformation that occurs in patients who embrace the prehab process. I've seen patients once debilitated by pain and inactivity regain their mobility and vitality. I've watched as individuals who struggled with obesity shed pounds and gained a new lease on life. I've marveled at the progress of diabetic patients who, through diligent management of their condition, stabilized their health to a point where surgery became a viable and safe option.

Following Dr. Watson's strategy, I've even had patients dance—literally dance—into their first post-op follow-up. This is the potential of a well-structured prehab program. It transforms the daunting and often discouraging process of preparing for surgery into a manageable and even empowering journey. This book is a testament to that potential, offering a clear, practical approach to prehabilitation that can change lives.

Those types of life-changing stories illustrate the profound impact that a well-thought-out prehabilitation strategy can have. Dr. Watson's approach is about more than just preparing for surgery; it's about supporting patients who take control of their health and well-being. It's about showing them that even in the face of complex medical challenges, there is a path forward.

In this book, Dr. Watson provides a comprehensive guide to prehabilitation that is both informative and inspiring. It's a resource that I recommend to my patients who are afflicted with various health issues. Whether they are dealing with joint pain, obesity, diabetes, or any other condition, this book offers practical strategies that can help them sidestep barriers to preparing for surgery and improving their overall quality of life.

To anyone reading this foreword, I urge you to take the principles in this book to heart. Embrace the prehab process. Follow the guidance provided, and commit to making the necessary changes. The journey may be challenging, but the rewards are immeasurable. You have the power to transform your health and set yourself up for a successful surgical outcome. With the help of Dr. Watson's roadmap, you can navigate the prehabilitation journey with confidence and achieve the best possible results.

INTRODUCTION

TAKING BACK CONTROL

"Three of the most difficult aspects of severe, chronic illness are the long waits, tough decisions, and financial struggles. Transcending these struggles requires the support and wisdom of family, friends, and medical personnel."
—FRANK LIGONS, CHRONIC ILLNESS SPEAKER AND ACTIVIST

THE WORLD IS FULL OF PEOPLE TRYING TO GET FROM ONE PLACE to another. Travel is an inevitable part of our existence, and we often find ourselves split down the middle, separated into two groups—drivers and passengers.

Individuals living with serious diagnoses are, in a way, similar to travelers on a busy interstate. If you picked up this book, you or a loved one might feel like a helpless passenger with no idea where you're going or control over how you'll get there. Your metaphorical car is wildly accelerating, hurtling toward that point where chronic disease or acute illness rears its head. Eventually, either of these could require major surgery or treatments that would be neither simple nor stress-free. Feelings of powerlessness during this are like a weight around your neck, sapping morale and draining quality of life.

Thankfully, an alternative exists. You're not destined to be the passenger in a vehicle careening toward the unknown. You likely sought out this guide because you or a loved one are likely facing an upcoming medical journey. Your interest in taking the preparation into your own hands is good news because this can potentially benefit you every step of the way. It hardly requires mental gymnastics to realize that like on any difficult expedition, modest preparation may pay enormous dividends.

In the case of any medical battle—anything from treatment for cancer to major joint replacement surgery—the weeks leading up to treatment are often anxiety-ridden and sleepless. However, individuals can choose to convert their inner tension into meaningful preparation. As an example, in some cases, the period prior to cancer treatment can be *so* productive and beneficial for outcomes that oncologists may recommend delaying surgical removal of cancer to invest time in physical therapy, nutritional optimization, and better chronic disease control. By improving physical resilience, patients tend to suffer fewer complications of treatment and have better outcomes. Maximizing benefit during this time before treatment is what prehabilitation is all about. And yes, it is actually that "simple."

"Simple" doesn't quite tell the whole story. The concepts and plans involved with prehabilitation (prehab) are straightforward, but the required effort is significant. To truly move the needle in a relatively short period of time, prehab programs require the immersion of a boot camp. This book serves as a guide and reference for what to expect throughout the most common medical journeys, with particular emphasis on prehab. The ultimate goal is returning to the best potential quality of life, and the few weeks of invested effort have the power to be life-changing.

WE COULD ALL USE A GUIDE

Just like prehab, this book was designed to be straightforward and useful. At its heart is an explanation of the core components (pillars) of an effective prehabilitation program, broken down into three categories—exercise, lifestyle, and the nervous system. Each contains its own concepts and their interventions. The three pillars complement a war chest of diagnostic tests and medications that might cross your path while working with your medical team. Finally, we apply this information in chapters dedicated to different medical scenarios—spine surgery and joint replacement, cancer treatment, bariatric surgery, amputations, transplantation, and a final combined chapter of fertility and gynecologic surgeries.

> Disclaimer: While the information within these pages can be helpful, it is presented for educational purposes. This book is not considered medical advice or medical treatment. Do not attempt to implement any aspect of this book without the recommendation of your personal medical provider. Your unique situation may differ from the scenarios presented in this book.

Instead, consider this your key to get back in the driver's seat. While this book isn't a replacement for personalized care, it details what may lie ahead, the terms your medical team may use, and low-risk interventions to discuss with your medical team—strategies like improving your sleep quality, ways to exercise for maximum benefit, and medications that may treat multiple illnesses at once. It also contains a peek behind the curtain into what medications and treatment options might become available in the near future.

Odds are, this is one of your first times hearing the term *prehab*. Or, if not, you'd at least get a few blank stares mentioning it in a crowded room. The premise behind prehabilitation acknowledges that the average person is not in their ideal health status. Life involves stress and busy schedules, which then lead to fast food during a few minutes of peace watching television. Exercise often falls by the wayside. Bad sleep and occasional happy hours only add insult to injury.

This is a reality many people face and is nothing to feel guilty about. Compounding these factors over time is why most people end up needing intensive intervention to get back on track. The following chapters serve to point out some healthy "nudges" to improve your baseline health. This is far from busywork just to kill time and redirect nervous energy before surgery—prehab creates actual, tangible benefits for many. When done correctly, a prehabilitation program can improve one's health such that when it "takes a hit" from major surgery, the individual is still better off than when they started. If we're discussing treatment for a *terminal* illness, prehab has the potential to make the person's remaining time better and longer.

OVER OR UNDER

Like the name suggests, prehab is all about what happens before major surgery or other intensive treatments begin. This comes with one last piece of context. Many chronic illnesses like high blood pressure and diabetes are associated with higher body weights. To address this, a large portion of the interventions in this book directly assist with weight loss. Although having a high body weight does not automatically mean poor health, the association is strong enough that "losing weight" may be the goal for a number of proposed concepts. This falls under the umbrella of *obesity medicine*, a term which is not pejorative but instead recognizes that obesity is a disease of which the medical establishment is gaining a better understanding and developing better treatments with broader health benefits.

The weight loss effort central in many prehab programs is far from a vanity push. For folks with overweight/obesity (this is the preferred terminology, instead of the outdated "obese patient" or "overweight patient"), research demonstrates that any weight loss before bariatric surgery is associated with a bonus of approximately 5 percent extra weight loss on top of what is normally expected from surgery.[1] Losing weight prior to abdominal surgeries, in particular, decreases the size of organs and effectively clears space in the abdomen. This makes the operation easier for the surgeons, which decreases the time required and may result in fewer complications. Optimizing control of diabetes *before* and *during* a surgical procedure is another critical intervention. This reduces the risk of infection at the incision by improving blood flow to the area and essentially lessening the amount of food (sugar) for bacteria to eat.[2]

In fact, research has shown that for patients with obesity, the more physically fit an individual is prior to surgery, the less likely they are to have medical complications within the first

---

[1] Masha Livhits et al., "Does Weight Loss Immediately before Bariatric Surgery Improve Outcomes: A Systematic Review," *Surgery for Obesity and Related Diseases* 5, no. 6 (November 2009): 717, https://doi.org/10.1016/j.soard.2009.08.014.

[2] Usama Iqbal et al., "Preoperative Patient Preparation in Enhanced Recovery Pathways," *Journal of Anaesthesiology Clinical Pharmacology* 35, Suppl. 1 (April 2019): S19, https://doi.org/10.4103/joacp.JOACP_54_18.

thirty days after surgery.[3] For patients with obesity who joined the study and also had weight-related chronic diseases like high blood pressure or diabetes, weight loss had a greater impact on lowering their risk of surgical complications. Patients who lost a given amount of weight with lifestyle changes and medication fared even better than those who lost the equivalent amount through bariatric surgery. Simply put, losing weight is often a major part of prehab and can have many benefits.

The concept of prehabilitation is becoming increasingly popular. The same research mentioned above proposed another great point. Some prehabilitation programs did not provide a significant benefit at all. Examining these individual programs, the theme is clear. A plan was likely to be of little benefit if the patient was not able to regularly or actively engage with *each* component (adherence with the program matters) or if the intervention was not comprehensive enough. The most effective programs included at least weekly meetings with specialists such as nutritionists, personal trainers or physical therapists, physicians, or psychologists. Dedication from a large team increased patients' commitment to the program and, given the diverse plan of attack, helped them accomplish a lot in limited available time. Effective prehab programs increase patient engagement.

Weight loss isn't the goal of *all* prehab programs. Patients who are underweight have their own shared health complications as well, especially before a major intervention. In these individuals, low body weight may contribute to *frailty*, a clinical term that generally refers to low body weight, low muscle mass, and increased risk of injury and illness.

---

[3] Natalie A. Smith et al., "Preoperative Assessment and Prehabilitation in Patients with Obesity Undergoing Non-Bariatric Surgery: A Systematic Review," *Journal of Clinical Anesthesia* 78 (June 2022): 1–15, 110676, https://doi.org/10.1016/j.jclinane.2022.110676.

One of the core goals of prehabilitation is to increase resilience regardless of starting body weight. This directly ties to better outcomes during and after surgery along with a lower chance of complications. Consider frailty to be the opposite of resilient. Some chronic diseases like cancer, lung diseases, and HIV/AIDS, among others, are associated with the condition *cachexia*, essentially frailty with an emphasis on the physical aspects of muscle wasting and loss of body mass. Optimizing the health of patients with frailty is similar to treating patients with obesity, although some of the supporting medication understandably involves stimulating appetite and reversing *catabolism*, or tissue breakdown.

PATIENT EDUCATION

Not only is this book a reference for prehabilitation programs in preparation for several types of medical interventions, but it prepares readers for what to expect throughout their medical journey. Knowledge is a tool that can help patients better advocate for themselves as well as better understand each stage of care.

Patient education offers many benefits to promote thriving throughout a successful major medical procedure timeline. For example, research suggests face-to-face education instead of written or video-based instruction prior to cancer surgery best improves presurgical anxiety and patient satisfaction.[4] Related research on preoperative education for colorectal cancer surgery showed improvements in the patients' recovery of "preopera-

---

4   Amy Waller et al., "Preparatory Education for Cancer Patients Undergoing Surgery: A Systematic Review of Volume and Quality of Research Output over Time," *Patient Education and Counseling* 98, no. 12 (December 2015): 1540–1549, https://doi.org/10.1016/j.pec.2015.05.008.

tive global health status," self-image, and even the length of hospital stays.[5]

Likely, taking some of the unknown out of the fight with cancer and building patient-provider trust contributed to the success and treatment satisfaction of these patients.[6] Using education to foster confidence may support patients when overcoming short-term setbacks by helping them maintain an overall long view.

PREPARING FOR PREHABILITATION

It might seem like overkill to prepare for a program that will then prepare you for a major medical intervention. Think of this as more of a mental preparation. It's easy to get lost in the wilderness when you or a loved one is overwhelmed by a diverse team of specialists, procedures, and new medications. Regardless of the medical battle, this can be downright intimidating.

The first purpose of this text is to act as a compass, pointing readers and their loved ones toward the finish line. Second, it provides a more detailed viewpoint to explain the purpose of those tests, treatments, and providers along the way. Each of these has a dedicated, condition-specific chapter to reference again when diving into what holds the most relevance to your personal journey.

The road ahead could be long and difficult. There may be setbacks or complications. But you remain in control of your

---

5 Lesley Larissa Koet et al., "Effectiveness of Preoperative Group Education for Patients with Colorectal Cancer: Managing Expectations," *Supportive Care in Cancer* 29, no. 9 (2021): 5263–5271, https://doi.org/10.1007/s00520-021-06072-5.

6 Mei-Yu Yeh et al., "The Relation between Patient Education, Patient Empowerment and Patient Satisfaction: A Cross-Sectional-Comparison Study," *Applied Nursing Research* 39 (February 2018): 11–17, https://doi.org/10.1016/j.apnr.2017.10.008.

mindset and your preparation. Don't ever think that there's nothing you can do. Prehabilitation offers a path forward that, if done correctly, can lead to better surgical outcomes, overall health, and quality of life.

PART I

CHAPTER 1

THE RECIPE FOR PREHABILITATION SUCCESS

THE SPARK FOR THE IDEA THAT GREW INTO MY PREHABILITAtion obsession first jolted me while working an overnight shift as an intern.

I was facing the prospect of "graduating" internship and proceeding to the remainder of my residency in physical medicine & rehabilitation. I finally knew enough about internal medicine to apply it within the context of the human body I found most interesting—muscles, bones, and the nervous system. Specifically, why after even a "routine" major surgery, patients who were once physically strong and independent seemed unexpectedly weak and dependent on others. Why was rehab necessary?

Eventually, I likened it to trying a complex exercise for the first time, like a pushup. I was a personal trainer in college, so naturally this was the language in which I thought. For a new exercise, you're typically limited by the weakest muscle—your weakest link in the chain. If you've got a strained muscle in your shoulder, it doesn't matter how strong your pecs are; you'll still be stuck lying face down. In the language of rehabilitation, all it takes is one link weakened by the surgery/illness or muscle atrophy after lying in a hospital bed for a week or two, and suddenly you require a "two-person assist" to get out of bed. This was epiphany number one.

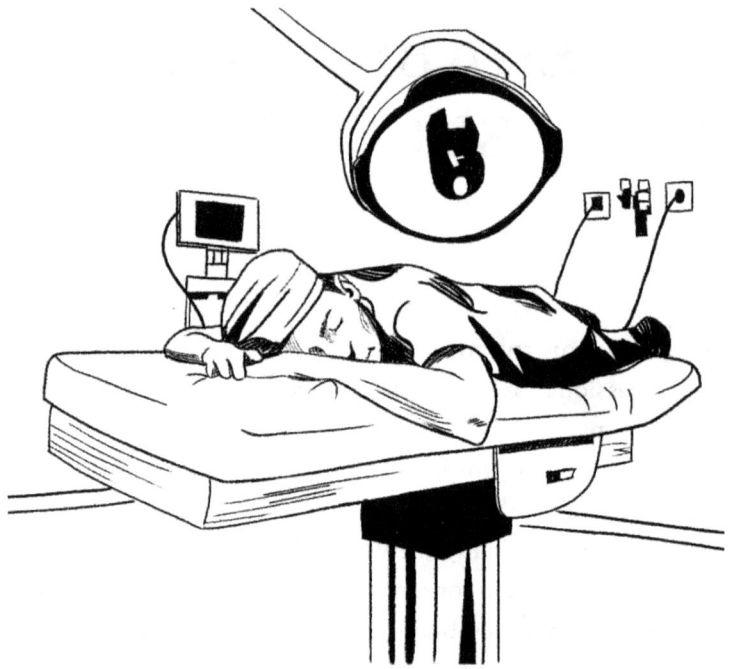

Artist's rendering of a night shift intern's happy place

Again, I was a trainer, and I knew how hard it was to coach someone into getting in shape. Even for the sake of "maintaining wellness" or staying healthy to play with his or her children, most clients still found life getting in the way because careers, hobbies, and those same kids took the understandable priority over a vaguely defined end point. An open-ended goal of "exercise three to four times per week, thirty to forty minutes per day...*forever*" can be hard to maintain because if you miss one day, well, you've got forever to make it up. Yet before a major elective procedure, you don't have forever. You've got a few months, max. Anyone can dig deep for a few weeks if there is a known payoff at the end, especially when the end is visible from the start.

No one said prehab would be easy, but I'm here to tell you that the growing body of research practically shouts it from the rooftops: prehab will be worth it. Whether you have three weeks or three months, there are positive changes that can affect your health prior to surgery, during surgery, and long after you've entered the recovery process.

Broadly, prehabilitation encompasses any pre-procedural lifestyle change. Things like starting a fitness program, quitting smoking, and transitioning to a protein-rich and processed-carb-restricted diet all fall under the prehab umbrella, but those barely scratch the surface.

Initiating an immersive boot camp-type program after receiving a life-changing diagnosis or enduring a decade of progressively worsening joint or back pain may feel like the furthest thing from ideal timing. After receiving such a diagnosis, patients are commonly overcome by a feeling of powerlessness. Likely, there are a million non-prehab things on their minds. However, this is the best time to get engaged and drive this thing instead of remaining a passenger along for the ride.

One of the most important things at this stage is to dig deep and find that willpower to dive headlong into an effective prehab program. For one, this makes the rest of the experience a lot less dehumanizing. Patient education is central in prehab, and that "cog in the wheel" sensation goes away when an individual has an understanding of what specialists they're seeing and why certain recommendations are made. Along with a sense of empowerment, staying engaged in the decision-making process has the potential to greatly improve outcomes.

BACK TO BASICS

Prehabilitation is full of common sense concepts, but in the general scope of healthcare, it's somewhat off the beaten path. While this is rapidly evolving, patients should familiarize themselves with the process, recurring themes, and key terms.

A physiatrist is a doctor who specializes in physical medicine & rehabilitation. These are board-certified rehab professionals, not just any doctors working in a rehab setting. For ease of terminology, your prehabilitation provider will be referred to as your physiatrist moving forward, though other informed providers may assume this role due to the scarcity of physiatrists. Prehab covers a lot of ground, often including several specialists, but your physiatrist is "riding shotgun" next to you on this journey, providing guidance throughout.

Your physiatrist will prescribe a diverse program designed with the right dose of each intervention to maximize impact and minimize discouragement during limited available time. In this phase, the physiatrist will identify areas (overall fitness level, nutrition, sleep, etc.) that will most meaningfully impact a patient's resilience. At the same time, he or she will lobby the other treating specialists to maximize time for these interventions. Obtaining the buy-in of other providers is becoming easier as, in most cases, surgeons and oncologists are studying the benefits of deliberately delaying treatment to allow time for prehabilitation.[7] Even in cases of newly identified cancer—a scenario in which most individuals would want to start treatment right away—research suggests that often the risk of worsening is low and the benefit from prehab can be significant. Some panels of surgical specialists now include prehabilitation for high-risk patients in their new guidelines for procedures within the umbrella of their specialty.[8]

In other words, the bottom-line goal for any procedure has always been better outcomes and fewer complications along the way, and prehabilitation is becoming increasingly accepted as a means to this end. But that doesn't mean prehab comes without its own unique challenges.

FINDING YOUR WHY

Stress isn't always bad for the body. Pain doesn't necessarily mean damage is being done. It's common, and understandable, for someone to avoid exercise on an arthritic joint because they're worried about causing further damage. However, exercise is one of the best sustainable remedies for bad arthritis pain by improving circulation of anti-inflammatory molecules. So similar to how exercise acutely raises heart rate but improves the cardiovascular system's function in the long term, exercise may stress a "bad" joint in the moment but improve pain moving

---

7   Anna Shukla et al., "Attitudes and Perceptions to Prehabilitation in Lung Cancer," *Integrative Cancer Therapies* 19 (2020): 1534735420924466, https://doi.org/10.1177/1534735420924466.

8   Timothy J. P. Batchelor et al., "Guidelines for Enhanced Recovery after Lung Surgery: Recommendations of the Enhanced Recovery after Surgery (ERAS) Society and the European Society of Thoracic Surgeons (ESTS)," *European Journal of Cardio-Thoracic Surgery* 55, no. 1 (January 2019): 91–115, https://doi.org/10.1093/ejcts/ezy301; Erik Stenberg et al., "Guidelines for Perioperative Care in Bariatric Surgery: Enhanced Recovery after Surgery (ERAS) Society Recommendations: A 2021 Update," *World Journal of Surgery* 46, no. 4 (April 2022): 729–751, https://doi.org/10.1007/s00268-021-06394-9.

forward because muscles strengthen and inflammation eases *cumulatively* after exercise. This effect may not last forever but should at least improve pain and stiffness until surgery provides a permanent fix. So when exercising safely, the corresponding pain may not originate from direct trauma. That's useful information when it comes to prehab.

An immersive program requiring dedicated focus provides an *active* waiting process prior to a surgery. Prehab programs are tailored to the individual, but they all require some form of activity to maximize benefits. This gives patients the opportunity to impact the outcome of their healthcare journey actively and meaningfully—the chance to regain control of their health and life's direction.

Yes, this might be difficult at times. Certain parts of a prehab program may not be everyone's definition of "fun." The less time a patient has before surgery or other treatments, the more intensive the program typically must be to create a true impact. Again, this requires high internal motivation. For some, a new diagnosis ignites this fire. Others require an external push to break through the initial paralysis, which is why some multidisciplinary clinics include specialized psychologists. Once invested, patients may then see the gradual benefits of their effort, like improved exercise tolerance, better chronic disease control, or simply less anxiety about their health.

Any of these can stoke the simmering motivational fire into a roaring blaze.

This describes *how* a patient finds their motivation for a prehab program in the face of a looming battle, but the *why* is just as inspiring for action. The research clearly demonstrates how potentially beneficial a pre-procedural "boot camp" can be for promoting quality of life during treatment and after completion. Based on the outcomes benefits alone, it wouldn't be surprising if insurance companies began outwardly *recommending* these plans (beyond simply reimbursing them) as a win for everyone involved. Digging deep and contributing the effort can go a long way for quality of life before and after treatment, plus better outcomes from treatment. Your why is personal, but these often boil down to wanting to live a better, healthier life with greater functional capabilities.

This is a good moment to include a preemptive answer to a reasonable concern: research suggests that delaying treatment for cancer by a few weeks for prehabilitation does not have a negative impact on rates of cancer recurrence or mortality at a population level.[9] On top of this, prehab can significantly increase muscle mass in this short period of time, which is important for conditions like cancer and bariatric surgery that may accelerate muscle loss. Building some physical reserves is important for the body and mind in these treatment situations. Possibly related to this resilience, a patient's hospitalization length of stay may decrease because of prehab.[10] However the "population level" may not perfectly represent every individual case, so this is a personal decision everyone receiving care must make with their individual treatment team.

These are the types of considerations patients should have prior to a major medical intervention. Even if their hospital doesn't offer a similar service, patients and caregivers should consider investing in a meal subscription to decrease cognitive

---

[9] Maud T. A. Strous et al., "Impact of Therapeutic Delay in Colorectal Cancer on Overall Survival and Cancer Recurrence—Is There a Safe Timeframe for Prehabilitation?," *European Journal of Surgical Oncology* 45, no. 12 (December 2019): 2295–2301, https://doi.org/10.1016/j.ejso.2019.07.009.

[10] James R. Bundred et al., "Prehabilitation prior to Surgery for Pancreatic Cancer: A Systematic Review," *Pancreatology* 20, no. 6 (September 2020): 1243–1250, https://doi.org/10.1016/j.pan.2020.07.411.

burden and ensure/maintain nutritional optimization.[11] Food is fuel, and how we fuel our bodies directly impacts prehab programs' success rates.

AVOIDING MISCONCEPTIONS

Any preparatory program before a medical intervention may get the "prehab" label slapped onto it. But the takeaway is that not every prehab program is created equal. Often, physical therapy or surgical practices will include select important components and be worth the effort. Others provide marginal benefits beyond finding an activity to occupy one's time and focus, which truthfully is better than nothing but leaves so many other potential benefits on the table. These at least give individuals with anticipatory anxiety a means of channeling that nervous energy into a potentially helpful activity, though the data don't support unanimous benefit for some of these types of programs. Effective prehabilitation is what we're after and what this book will illustrate.

In most cases, ineffective programs share similar characteristics: they are often too short (less than one month), leave too much ambiguity for patient interpretation, lack personalization to individuals' abilities, and do not include multiple sessions (of physical therapy, dietician counseling, physician counseling, etc.) in each week. Generally, if it *feels* too easy, the program probably isn't all that effective. However, this doesn't mean a prehab program must be difficult. A good rule of thumb is the shorter the program, the more intense it must be to effect change.

---

[11] Vera E. IJmker-Hemink et al., "Effect of a Preoperative Home-Delivered, Protein-Rich Meal Service to Improve Protein Intake in Surgical Patients: A Randomized Controlled Trial," *Journal of Parenteral and Enteral Nutrition* 45, no. 3 (March 2021): 479–489, https://doi.org/10.1002/jpen.2015.

Programs that are less than one month can absolutely promote a benefit, but these will likely require higher weekly intensity of training and tighter control of nutritional parameters.

We must maximize the use of time before treatment. This often leads to a challenging program, but a benefit of prehab is that it's very much a defined and finite program. In that short amount of time, we're trying to incorporate tolerable exercise, implement a well-controlled diet, dramatically improve sleep quality, and address mood issues, to name a few priorities. That culminates in a multi-tiered, intensive regimen where the best mindset is often: *Dig down deep and get through these six weeks, and I'll be very much better for it.* You'll look back and admire all you accomplished.

THE THREE PILLARS OF PREHABILITATION

Roughly, prehabilitation is any pre-procedural health-optimizing intervention. Like any other treatment intended for health benefit, the determining factor is *dose*. In the context of exercise, dose is determined by frequency, intensity, type, and time spent participating. For dietary changes, dose implies the balance of macronutrients (protein, carbohydrates, and fat), which determines total calories, how they are divided throughout the day and week, and the other nutrients within the diet. When it comes to medications, well, dose is fairly self-evident.

Prehabilitation encompasses a diverse set of potential changes. Although there is no single authority on how prehab is defined, my colleagues and I typically break down the critical components of any effective program into three pillars: exercise, lifestyle, and neuropsychiatric (nervous system-related targets like sleep, mood, and pain).

Because of the exercise involved and the deconditioned (out-of-shape) state in which most of us live as a consequence of busy lives, the first stage of pre-procedural health optimization is after *screening*. This book, again, is *not medical advice*, but a safe piece of advice is to consult your personal physician prior to engaging in a new exercise program. The same illnesses that often require medical intervention also predispose individuals to other diseases that might quickly worsen when stressed with a new exercise program.

THE EXERCISE PILLAR

The American College of Sports Medicine provides guidelines for safely beginning exercise.[12] The following summary is not 100 percent comprehensive but reviews the most up-to-date suggestions at the time of this writing. First, individuals not currently participating in regular exercise should absolutely get pre-exercise clearance if they have known or suspected heart, lung, kidney, or metabolic (diabetes, blood pressure, or cholesterol) disease. After receiving clearance, they may begin with light to moderate intensity exercise and should only progress to greater intensity if able to complete the initial exercises without concerning symptoms such as chest discomfort (especially with exertion), shortness of breath or fatigue with mild to no exertion, dizziness, or fainting. Should these symptoms arise, individuals should immediately stop the exercise and consult medical attention.

Many of the procedures that benefit from prehabilitation, such as heart surgery, lung surgery, and chemotherapy, or extended bed rest negatively impact cardiopulmonary (heart/

---

12 Deborah Riebe et al., "Updating ACSM's Recommendations for Exercise Preparticipation Health Screening," *Medicine & Science in Sports & Exercise* 47, no. 11 (November 2015): 2473–2479, https://doi.org/10.1249/MSS.0000000000000664.

lung) function.[13] With this, we introduce a primary goal of the exercise pillar: improving cardiopulmonary or aerobic capacity. Here's an often misunderstood concept: aerobic benefits of exercise are not primarily from improved heart or lung function. Most of the benefit comes from muscles becoming more efficient at using the oxygen and fuel they have received. This is actually a better scenario, as it allows individuals with irreversible cardiopulmonary disease to obtain appreciable benefit from exercise.

Resistance (strength) training is the other half of the exercise picture, as the same negative forces of chemotherapy, surgery, and bed rest that affect aerobic capacity also quickly "burn away" muscle. Some degree of muscle loss is inevitable even in situations of intentional weight loss such as after bariatric surgery or using new, highly effective weight loss medications like semaglutide (Wegovy and Ozempic) or tirzepatide (Mountjaro and Zepbound).

Which type of exercise is best for a short-duration prehabilitation program? The glib answer is "Whichever one a patient will do." This is the most important part; if there is a type of exercise that motivates someone to regularly participate, *that* is the best type. Given multiple choices, the ideal combination is to emphasize variety. Combining aerobic and resistance training can maximize the benefits of building muscle with improved aerobic capacity. In this discussion, "aerobic training" includes various training styles from jogging at a steady pace to intervals of alternating high and low intensity and everything in between.

---

13   John Knight, Yamni Nigam, and Aled Jones, "Effects of Bedrest 1: Introduction and the Cardiovascular System," *Nursing Times*, November 26, 2018, https://www.nursingtimes.net/clinical-archive/cardiovascular-clinical-archive/effects-of-bedrest-1-introduction-and-the-cardiovascular-system-26-11-2018/; John Knight, Yamni Nigam, and Aled Jones, "Effects of Bedrest 1: Respiratory Haematologial Systems," *Nursing Times*, January 2, 2019, https://www.nursingtimes.net/clinical-archive/respiratory-clinical-archive/effects-of-bedrest-2-respiratory-and-haematological-systems-02-01-2019/.

Basic Types of Exercise Training:

TRAINING	DESCRIPTION
Resistance	The use of resistance to muscular contraction, typically measured with a defined set of repetitions (one, three, five, eight, etc.) to build strength and size of skeletal muscles with different techniques like free weights, machines, elastic bands, or bodyweight exercises.
Aerobic	Activities involving sustained work often measured over a time period (e.g., walking, cycling, running) and may be divided into two methodologies: Continuous (isokinetic), characterized by long-duration sessions performed at a continuous pace without rest. Intervals may be composed of short (e.g., four minutes), high-intensity bouts interspersed with active recovery (e.g., three minutes) at a lower intensity. This cycle is typically repeated at least three to four times per session. Inherently, higher intensity intervals are shorter in duration.
Balance	Movements to improve control of muscles responsible for standing upright like the core and legs. These are important for fall prevention.
Flexibility	Movements for improving mobility of muscles/tendons and the joints they control and maintaining full freedom of movement. This full range of motion helps eliminate inefficient, awkward movements and may indirectly reduce risk of injury.

A discussion of exercise therapies is incomplete without aquatherapy. Aquatherapy is a relatively under-the-radar means of physical activity that combines some of the best parts of exercise—resistance training, aerobic fitness, and social interaction—with the added benefit of reducing the normal heat-related discomfort of exercise. Plus, the water literally warms up muscles before exercise, and the buoyancy effect reduces weight on uncomfortable arthritic joints. In some rehabilitation studies, aquatherapy ranks highest in benefits over land-based activities for patients with obesity within domains like overall pain (outside of therapy sessions) and maladaptive behaviors to minimize activity-related painful movements.[14] In other words, aquatherapy further opens the door to participation in other exercise therapies.

Lift Lighter for Bigger Muscles?

Pain perception is often a huge limiting/modifying factor when it comes to starting or progressing a workout routine, especially when lifting relatively heavy weights. For experienced individuals, the inclination with painful joints, necks, and backs is to continue to increase the weight being lifted but limit the range of motion as a means of continuing progress while avoiding injury.

In reality, the opposite appears to be true. Muscles receive the greatest stimulus to grow and get stronger at the "stretch" portion of the repetition. For example, when performing a chest press-type exercise, muscles respond best to the tension on them when the weight has you feeling a stretch and your elbows are bent (as demonstrated below), *not* when your arms are fully extended in front of you.[15]

---

14 Joseph G. Wasser et al., "Exercise Benefits for Chronic Low Back Pain in Overweight and Obese Individuals," PM & R 9, no. 2 (February 2017): 181–192, https://doi.org/10.1016/j.pmrj.2016.06.019.

15 Shigeru Sato et al., "Elbow Joint Angles in Elbow Flexor Unilateral Resistance Exercise Training Determine Its Effects on Muscle Strength and Thickness of Trained and Non-Trained Arms," Frontiers in Physiology 12 (2021): 734509, https://doi.org/10.3389/fphys.2021.734509; Michal Krzysztofik et al., "Maximizing Muscle Hypertrophy: A Systematic Review of Advanced Resistance Training Techniques and Methods," International Journal of Environmental Research in Public Health 16, no. 24 (2019): 4897, https://doi.org/10.3390/ijerph16244897.

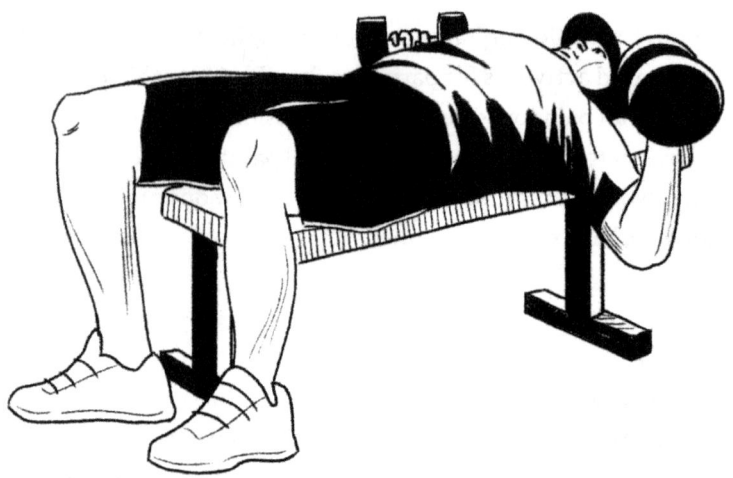

Example of appropriate depth for repetitions when performed with slow, controlled technique

When it comes to safety and injury prevention, controlling the weight as you are entering that stretch (the "eccentric" portion of the exercise) is critical for both preventing injury at that time and also increasing the stability and resilience of that joint and the tendons involved. By performing these in a repetition ("rep") range of approximately eight to twenty repetitions to near failure with slow, controlled eccentric movements, you will actually build *more* muscle, increase strength, and lower your risk of injury, even when compared with picking up a heavier weight that you can move fairly quickly through a narrower range of motion.[16] You'll also likely recover faster because the lower weight may be less taxing to your whole body. So you'll build muscle where you want without needlessly fatiguing the rest of your body.

---

16 Daniel E. Newmire and Darryn S. Willoughby, "Partial Compared with Full Range of Motion Resistance Training for Muscle Hypertrophy: A Brief Review and an Identification of Potential Mechanisms," *The Journal of Strength and Conditioning Research* 32, no. 9 (September 2018): 2652–2664, https://doi.org/10.1519/JSC.0000000000002723.

Related research will make your workouts simpler in other ways too. Instead of incorporating four or five exercises per muscle group (if you are feeling ambitious), two or three exercises done this way may actually give you better results. To maximize this benefit, you should nearly reach "failure"—the point at which you truly couldn't perform an additional repetition—in most of these sets. If you are nearly reaching failure, you couldn't possibly attack a group of muscles with a half dozen exercises, and you won't even need to. Two or three exercises performed well can be more than enough. So to continue the earlier example, a machine chest press of three sets of eight reps, followed by chest flys on a machine and finished with pushups (regular, knee pushups, or incline pushups with your feet on a bench if you are particularly well trained) could be a solid regimen to more than adequately work your pectoral, triceps, and deltoid muscles. Don't worry about varying this substantially from day to day either. You can perform the same exercises for a few weeks and continue to derive benefit. However, if you'd like some variety, that's fine as well. If you're making your sets count, the exact exercise is less important. Just make sure the movements are "compound" (multi-joint) movements like chest presses, shoulder presses, rows, squats, etc., instead of single joint movements like curls. The goal is to get the maximum benefit in the least amount of time with the lowest risk of injury.

Blood-Flow Restriction Training

Blood-flow restriction (BFR) training, also known as *kaatsu*, is a training style that essentially uses biochemistry to "trick" muscles into stimulating recovery as if they've lifted substantially heavier weight during strength training. Perform BFR with the guidance of a specialist, but for the sake of educational purposes, begin by applying a restrictive cuff around a limb closer to the body than the muscle that is performing work. For example, apply the cuff at the knee or thigh prior to doing calf raises for rehabbing a strained Achilles tendon. The amount of pressure should be enough to restrict blood from leaving the muscle, but it should be loose enough that arterial blood flow *into* the muscle continues. This is a tricky balance to achieve and another reason why BFR training requires the guidance of a specialist.

When utilizing BFR during resistance training, perform exercises beginning with a weight that is approximately one-quarter of your "one rep maximum" (1RM), which is the weight at which you can perform the exercise for only a single repetition. Most non-powerlifters have never determined their 1RM for various strength exercises, so alternatively, just choose a weight that feels quite light at first. Then, perform the exercise for fifteen to thirty repetitions as tolerated. Adjust the weight so that you reach failure in the fifteen-to-thirty-rep range. Some will instead use BFR to increase the difficulty of aerobic training if their pace or available time is limited by external factors.

There are a few important points to note regarding this practice. BFR is more difficult than it likely sounds. The same metabolic products—like lactate and acidic ions (H+)—that tell muscles to grow after exercise also create discomfort as they build up.[17] By preventing veins from carrying these compounds away, your muscles will be *unambiguously* aware of the exercise you're performing. This can be quite humbling given the reduced weight provoking this level of discomfort.

Another crucial point for novices is to keep the BFR cuffs

---

[17] Melissa C. Minniti et al., "The Safety of Blood Flow Restriction Training as a Therapeutic Intervention for Patients with Musculoskeletal Disorders: A Systematic Review," *The American Journal of Sports Medicine* 48, no. 7 (2020): 1773–1785, https://doi.org/10.1177/0363546519882652.

in place for limited periods of time. A general rule of thumb is to maintain pressure only during workout sets for resistance training, or for about fifteen to twenty minutes at a time for aerobic training. Prolonged restriction risks injury to the muscle, development of a blood clot, or other injury to blood vessels.[18] Some experienced individuals may exceed this time limit, but be cautious and, like everything else included in this book, seek guidance from a professional who knows your medical history.

There is no one situation where BFR is most useful. After open heart surgery, individuals are restricted from lifting more than a few pounds with their arms. Alternatively, an arthritic joint may not like movement while holding *any* weight, let alone anything resembling a 1RM. Individuals with advanced lung disease are also restricted in the weight they can lift, lest they overburden their heart and cause permanent damage. Cancer that has metastasized to bones increases the risk that these bones may break under heavy stress, even indirectly. For example, a spinal vertebra with multiple myeloma or prostate cancer metastases may be at risk of collapse with upper-body resistance training.

BFR allows individuals with any of these conditions—and others—to start or continue exercise training in order to adequately challenge their muscles. Even isometric exercises—holding a position without moving—quickly become challenging maneuvers even for the experienced athlete with the application of BFR cuffs.

The caveat is that current BFR programs likely didn't account for these types of advanced chronic diseases in their design. It's possible that available data could underestimate the potential

---

18 Stephen D. Patterson et al., "Blood Flow Restriction Exercise: Considerations of Methodology, Application, and Safety," *Frontiers in Physiology* 10 (2019): 533, https://doi.org/10.3389/fphys.2019.00533.

for adverse events in individuals with multiple vascular (blood vessels) or neuromuscular (nerves/muscles) comorbidities—the simultaneous presence of two or more medical conditions or diseases. On the other hand, however, this is the population who may benefit most from BFR as an introduction to exercise.

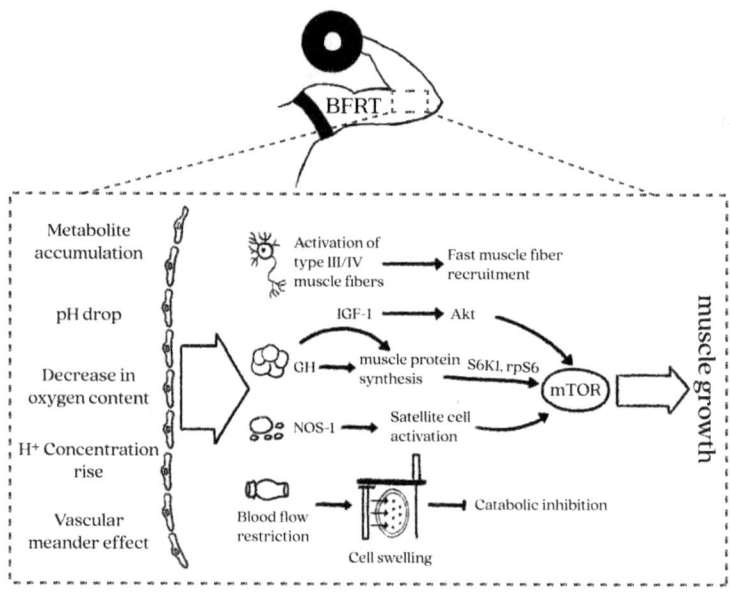

Deep dive into the mechanisms of how blood-flow restriction training (BFRT) stimulates muscle growth

In studies of patients with obesity, BFR resulted in higher metabolic demand despite low *perceived* exertion. This included significantly higher heart rate, oxygen consumption, and a 20.5 percent and 11 percent increase in energy expenditure in males and female participants, respectively.[19] Higher rates of adverse

---

19 Murat Karabulut and Sonio D. Garcia, "Hemodynamic Responses and Energy Expenditure during Blood Flow Restriction Exercise in Obese Population," *Clinical Physiology and Functional Imaging* 37, no. 1 (January 2017): 1–7, https://doi.org/10.1111/cpf.12258.

events weren't exhibited, meaning individuals with advanced chronic diseases may be safe to attempt BFR under strict supervision (and after receiving medical clearance). In summary, BFR can help bypass weight-bearing restrictions for resistance training or exercise tolerance affected by advanced chronic diseases.

High-Intensity Interval Training

High-intensity interval training (HIIT) alternates short periods of intense or explosive exercise with less intense recovery periods. This differs from aerobic training because the high level of intensity, interval duration, and number of repetitions forces the body to rely on anaerobic energy systems, breaking down glucose (blood sugar) without directly using oxygen.

A good way to think of HIIT is spurts of near-maximum effort sandwiched between active recovery time. Note that a recovery period is not a rest period. An example HIIT workout might alternate sprinting and light jogging. HIIT workouts can also incorporate cardiovascular activity and resistance training at the same time, with the key being triggering anaerobic energy production.

If this doesn't sound like fun, you're not alone. HIIT crams a lot of hard work into a relatively short period of time, making it quite efficient for reaching certain goals. Efficiency is our friend when conducting prehab because in most cases, time is limited.

Exercise Tailored to Metabolic Disease

Exercise and dietary intervention (which we'll discuss next in the lifestyle pillar) directly benefit an individual by improving blood pressure, cholesterol levels, and diabetes, but they have further compounded benefits. These measures facilitate weight loss, which can potentially trigger a positive feedback loop, making ongoing interventions even more effective.

Weight loss does not have to be substantial in individuals with high BMI (i.e., Class III obesity) to demonstrate improvements in obesity-related comorbidities for many. A 5 percent reduction in body weight can lead to significant improvements in:[20]

- Blood pressure
- Osteoarthritis symptoms
- Polycystic ovarian syndrome (PCOS)
- Gastroesophageal reflux disease (GERD) in women
- High cholesterol and triglycerides in the blood

A greater than 7 percent body weight reduction can further lower the risk of type 2 diabetes, and at least a 10 percent reduction in body weight can improve obstructive sleep apnea (OSA) and nonalcoholic fatty liver disease (NAFLD) or metabolic dysfunction-associated steatotic liver disease (MASLD).[21]

---

20 Judith E. Neter et al., "Influence of Weight Reduction on Blood Pressure: A Meta-Analysis of Randomized Controlled Trials," *Hypertension* 42, no. 5 (2003): 878–884, https://doi.org/10.1161/01.HYP.0000094221.86888.AE; Robin Christensen et al., "Effect of Weight Reduction in Obese Patients Diagnosed with Knee Osteoarthritis: A Systematic Review and Meta-Analysis," *Annals of the Rheumatic Diseases* 66, no. 4 (2007): 433–439, https://doi.org/10.1136/ard.2006.065904; J. Aaboe et al., "Effects of an Intensive Weight Loss Program on Knee Joint Loading in Obese Adults with Knee Osteoarthritis," *Osteoarthritis and Cartilage* 19, no. 7 (July 2011): 822–828, https://doi.org/10.1016/j.joca.2011.03.006; S. K. Graff et al., "Effects of Orlistat vs. Metformin on Weight Loss-Related Clinical Variables in Women with PCOS: Systematic Review and Meta-Analysis," *The International Journal of Clinical Practice* 70, no. 6 (2016): 450–461, https://doi.org/10.1111/ijcp.12787; N. de Bortoli et al., "Voluntary and Controlled Weight Loss Can Reduce Symptoms and Proton Pump Inhibitor Use and Dosage in Patients with Gastroesophageal Reflux Disease: A Comparative Study," *Diseases of the Esophagus* 29 (2016): 197–204, https://doi.org/10.1111/dote.12319.

21 David W. Hudgel et al., "The Role of Weight Management in the Treatment of Adult Obstructive Sleep Apnea: An Official American Thoracic Society Clinical Practice Guideline," *American Journal of Respiratory and Critical Care Medicine* 198, no. 6 (2018): e70–e87, https://doi.org/10.1164/rccm.201807-1326ST; Dimitrios A. Koutoukidis et al., "The Effect of the Magnitude of Weight Loss on Non-Alcoholic Fatty Liver Disease: A Systematic Review and Meta-Analysis," *Metabolism* 115 (February 2021): 154455, https://doi.org/10.1016/j.metabol.2020.154455.

For a two hundred fifty-pound individual, this is approximately nineteen and twenty-five pounds, respectively.

Aerobic exercise and resistance training in tandem have the potential to improve insulin sensitivity, the latter by increasing glucose storage capacity through hypertrophy—building muscles. Our muscles store glucose (sugar), so having more muscle volume is beneficial for individuals with diabetes.

Although exercise research is mixed, current research supports a general strategy of aerobic training with roughly a sustained heart rate of approximately 120 to 135 BPM (70–80 percent of maximum heart rate, calculated by subtracting the person's age from 220) for a fifty-year-old.[22] Another estimate for moderate intensity is using the talk test—you could *talk* but not *sing*. Evenly dividing these sessions so that an individual participates in aerobic activity approximately every forty-eight hours can sustain short-term diabetes-reversing effects.

A lack of available leisure time is often the limiting factor in exercise participation. A regimen that incorporates higher-intensity, lower-volume aerobic training frees up more time for resistance training. Paired resistance and aerobic training has the ability to achieve improvements in diabetes/prediabetes with much less required weight loss (approximately 3 percent). This lowers the risk of developing type 2 diabetes.[23]

---

[22] Vagner R. R. Silva et al., "The Effects of Ninety Minutes per Week of Moderate Intensity Aerobic Exercise on Metabolic Health in Individuals with Type 2 Diabetes: A Pilot Study," *Journal of Rehabilitation Therapy* 2, no. 2 (2020): 1–12, https://www.rehabiljournal.com/articles/the-effects-of-ninety-minutes-per-week-of-moderate-intensity-aerobic-exercise-on-metabolic-health-in-individuals-with-type-2-diabetes-a-pilot-study.pdf.

[23] Damon L. Swift et al., "Effects of Aerobic Training with and without Weight Loss on Insulin Sensitivity and Lipids," *PLoS One* 13, no. 5 (2018): 1–15, e0196637, https://doi.org/10.1371/journal.pone.0196637.

Prescribing Exercise

Realistic goals are important in the shared decision-making process. You're more likely to exercise and keep exercising if you (relatively) enjoy what you're doing and reach milestones along the way. Conversely, you're less likely to feel burned out or unmotivated if your goals are realistic, especially if they're shared with a physical or occupational therapist. Goals also serve as therapy endpoints that allow for informed modifications to the day-to-day plan based on progress.

Further, be aware of true exercise "stop signals." These include chest pain from exertion, proximal extremity pain (nearer to the center of the body or point of attachment), nausea, feeling faint, or inappropriate musculoskeletal pain. Also be aware of "caution" signals like excessive breathlessness that indicate a need to dial down the intensity. Many of these signs/symptoms are subjective, so personalized counseling on normal fatigue versus moderate flag symptoms must be discussed with one's physician.

Incorporating exercise in its various forms is critical to an effective prehab program. Keep in mind, however, that exercise is one pillar in a trio of necessary intervention categories. The pillars work together; one won't be as effective or complete without the other two. With that said, the next pillar focuses on the bulk of our health optimization that can have a huge impact on quality of life and good outcomes.

THE LIFESTYLE PILLAR

The second pillar is all about a patient's lifestyle, specifically most of the interventions that have the potential to improve health outside of an exercise setting. A major prehab goal is to improve the rate of recovery after surgery, but the sooner someone starts making healthy lifestyle changes, the better off they'll be. In part, that means that this pillar is especially about a better quality of life right now.

Some of the most important lifestyle changes a person can make to improve their health are right in front of our faces, and these often comprise formal "enhanced recovery after surgery" programs. ERAS protocols list quitting smoking, reducing or eliminating alcohol consumption, and losing weight (or gaining muscle if frailty is a concern) as three impactful things someone can do to prepare for surgery. It's no secret that smoking, drinking alcohol, and excessive weight gain take a toll on our bodies, and giving them up is clearly a cornerstone of any effective prehab program.

Removing smoking from your lifestyle is quite possibly the single most effective thing a patient can do to improve their surgical outcome as well as long-term health status. Smoking cessation moves the needle the most when it comes to health improvement prior to surgery, and it likely makes the biggest impact long after surgery or treatment. But it isn't quite that simple because there's some timing at play. Smoking cessation can be followed by one to two weeks of worse respiratory function.[24] Think of quitting smoking like fighting a bad illness—sometimes you have to get worse before you get better. This means that it isn't a good idea to quit *right* before a major surgery.

If a four-week time period allows, a patient should quit smoking immediately and receive resources to resolve any adverse symptoms prior to their procedure. A study conducted

---

[24] M. Ussher et al., "Increase in Common Cold Symptoms and Mouth Ulcers Following Smoking Cessation," *Tobacco Control* 12, no. 1 (2003): 86–88, https://doi.org/10.1136/tc.12.1.86.

specifically for cancer-treatment preparation used a four-week cessation period prior to starting chemotherapy without any related negative effects.[25] When done in tandem with other lifestyle interventions and our exercise and neuropsychiatric pillars, it plays an important role in better outcomes and improved quality of life. Plus, some find it easier to sustain a major behavioral change when paired with other similar changes—think quitting drinking alcohol *and* smoking simultaneously instead of sequentially.

Essentially, everything in prehab that isn't related to exercise, the brain, or peripheral nervous system falls under our "lifestyle" pillar. That means this pillar is diverse and wide ranging, but it's also extremely important. Each pillar alone offers benefits, but combining all three offers the most potential improvement.

Nutritional Considerations

Optimizing nutrition is crucial on its own, but the real magic is how it can aid exercise. If you think of the body like a machine, fuel absolutely matters. Proper nutrition yields faster improvement of metabolic markers, improved healing from surgery or treatment, and even greater resilience to trauma in the brain or spinal cord.[26]

However, of all areas of "medical science," nutrition may be the least generalizable. People and their bodily needs differ, and landing on the "best" diet for short- and long-term wellness

---

[25] Shintaro Tarumi et al., "Pulmonary Rehabilitation During Induction Chemoradiotherapy for Lung Cancer Improves Pulmonary Function," *The Journal of Thoracic and Cardiovascular Surgery* 149, no. 2 (February 2015): 569–573, https://doi.org/10.1016/j.jtcvs.2014.09.123.

[26] Jessica N. Holland and Adam T. Schmidt, "Static and Dynamic Factors Promoting Resilience Following Traumatic Brain Injury: A Brief Review," *Neural Plasticity* 2015, no. 1 (January 2015): 4–5, 902802, https://doi.org/10.1155/2015/902802.

is a lot like confidently decreeing the best type of shoe. Obviously, the purpose of that shoe matters, unless you're the kind of person who squats in high heels or goes jogging in bowling shoes. Nutritional research constantly revises what is considered "best," and these studies often have unaccounted-for variables that can unexpectedly impact the outcomes. Further, the ideal diet for someone with frailty is very different from that of someone with obesity and diabetes, hence the need for personalization.

We aren't interested in a mythical "perfect diet," but a few solid nutritional concepts can serve as lasting guidelines for prehabilitation and simplify meal prep decisions.

Clinical research is increasingly suggesting that fructose, or "fruit sugar," contributes significantly to metabolic disease. Unless lessened by high dietary fiber, such as when eaten within fruit, ingesting more than roughly three to four grams of fructose in one sitting overwhelms the intestine's inherent ability to shield the liver from its negative effects.[27] After absorption, fructose heads to the liver and can negatively affect insulin sensitivity, energy storage, and downstream metabolic comorbidities like gout.

Health professionals have known for a long time that fructose consumption is a risk factor for elevated uric acid and gout attacks. In addition, recent studies have linked uric acid to mitochondrial dysfunction (i.e., worse calorie burning and energy production), high blood pressure, and kidney disease.[28] There's a

---

[27] Cholsoon Jang et al., "The Small Intestine Converts Dietary Fructose into Glucose and Organic Acids," *Cell Metabolism* 27, no. 2 (2018): 351–361.e3, https://doi.org/10.1016/j.cmet.2017.12.016.

[28] Laura G. Sanchez-Lozada et al., "Uric Acid and Hypertension: An Update with Recommendations," *American Journal of Hypertension* 33, no. 7 (July 2020): 583–594, https://doi.org/10.1093/ajh/hpaa044.

biological drive to accumulate fat stores for unexpected famine. Modern humans in a nutrient-dense environment must exercise significant restraint against this, since fructose is often added to foods to enhance taste. A simple takeaway is to eat fructose in limited amounts and only when it's packaged in fiber-rich fruits.

If your takeaway from all that was "excess sugar is bad," then you're on the right track. For prehab and general health purposes, place an emphasis on avoiding sugar-sweetened beverages like sodas, sweet teas, and juices, and minimize consuming fruits with high sugar and low fiber, such as grapes, mangos, and figs. This doesn't mean an optimized diet must cut out everything sweet. Individuals craving sugar can eat relatively low-fructose/sugar fruits like berries, citrus fruits, and kiwi. Similarly, switch from sugar-sweetened beverages to artificially sweetened beverages to further reduce excess sugar in the diet.

Regarding artificial sweeteners, research is confirming that they alter the microbiota (the microorganisms found within all complex life) in rodents.[29] New data even suggests that sweeteners saccharin and sucralose may impact insulin sensitivity, so it can't be said that artificial sweeteners don't come with their own potential drawbacks.[30] But transitioning from sugar to artificial sweeteners is a "harm reduction" technique. If the alternative is high-fructose corn syrup or sucrose, calorie-free sweeteners are undoubtedly a positive substitute, especially during short periods during prehabilitation.[31]

---

29 Jotham Suez et al., "Artificial Sweeteners Induce Glucose Intolerance by Altering the Gut Microbiota," *Nature* 514, no. 7521 (2014): 181–186, https://doi.org/10.1038/nature13793.

30 Jotham Suez et al., "Personalized Microbiome-Driven Effects of Non-Nutritive Sweeteners on Human Glucose Tolerance," *Cell* 185, no. 18 (2022): 3307–3328, https://doi.org/10.1016/j.cell.2022.07.016.

31 Karl Z. Nadolsky, "Counterpoint: Artificial Sweeteners for Obesity—Better Than Sugary Alternatives; Potentially a Solution," *Endocrine Practice* 27, no. 10 (October 2021): 1056–1061, https://doi.org/10.1016/j.eprac.2021.06.013.

From there, a logical next step is understanding supplements that can enhance a healthy, low-sugar diet.

The Power of Supplements

Supplementation can be a powerful and relatively easy way to potentially make a noticeable difference in a person's health. Dietary supplements provide extra nutrients, vitamins, and minerals to complement daily nutrition. Simply put, a person experiencing malnutrition, or lacking certain nutrients the body needs for proper function, isn't going to be able to prepare as effectively during prehab. Diet deficiencies or insufficiencies may make other interventions less effective or may slow recovery from exercise.

To determine what supplements may be beneficial, the prehab team examines a patient for signs of malnutrition and deficiencies. This includes questioning about sensory disturbances that could indicate neuropathy (malfunctioning nerves), fatigue that could suggest anemia (low red blood cell count "quality"), and any restrictive eating patterns that increase risk for nutrient deficiency. In individuals pursuing bariatric surgery, these history questions or a screening using specific blood tests are typically standard, as any starting deficiencies have the potential to worsen immediately after surgery.[32]

Even for individuals without any deficiencies, basic supplementation can accelerate recovery from exercise and ultimately surgery, build muscle mass, and even improve overall physical resilience.

---

32 Leigh A. Peterson et al., "Vitamin D Status and Supplementation Before and After Bariatric Surgery: A Comprehensive Literature Review," *Surgery for Obesity and Related Diseases* 12, no. 3 (March 2016): 693–702, https://doi.org/10.1016/j.soard.2016.01.001.

Creatine

One universally beneficial supplement is creatine, often sold as creatine monohydrate. Athletes have used creatine for decades to improve muscle mass and physical performance, which means creatine is one of the most extensively studied performance supplements available.

Creatine comes naturally from meat products in our diets, and our livers and kidneys also produce it in small amounts. Creatine is a source of cellular energy, largely in muscle cells, but it is also used in other metabolically active tissue like the central nervous system.[33]

One common rumor about creatine is that it causes water retention, which is clinically meaningful to people with kidney and heart disease that make them sensitive to changes in fluid balance. But that rumor doesn't tell the entire story. In reality, studies show that fluid volume in the body increases when a person starts taking creatine. This is more common if the regimen is "loaded" with several days of extremely high doses to spur faster uptake by muscles.[34] However, over time, this fluid redistributes, suggesting low risk of complications in most people.

Another unfounded concern is that creatine and protein supplementation can cause or contribute to worsening kidney disease. Protein's role in this area isn't straightforward and will be discussed later, but when it comes to creatine, this rumor is completely untrue. This misconception is likely the result of

---

[33] Robert H. Andres et al., "Functions and Effects of Creatine in the Central Nervous System," *Brain Research Bulletin* 76, no. 4 (2008): 329–343, https://doi.org/10.1016/j.brainresbull.2008.02.035.

[34] Rebecca M. Lopez et al., "Does Creatine Supplementation Hinder Exercise Heat Tolerance or Hydration Status? A Systematic Review with Meta-Analyses," *Journal of Athletic Training* 44, no. 2 (2009): 215–223, https://doi.org/10.4085/1062-6050-44.2.215.

the way kidney function is traditionally measured.[35] *Creatinine* is a byproduct that comes from the breakdown of creatine in the body. All else held equal, healthcare professionals interpret a rise in creatinine as worsened kidney function. However, this doesn't take into account people who use creatine supplements. As creatine levels increase from outside sources, so does the metabolism of creatine into creatinine. This has nothing to do with decreased kidney function and everything to do with higher total body levels of creatine, which becomes correlated with an increase in skeletal muscle.

Resistance training and muscle growth are important parts of prehab—as introduced in the exercise pillar—and creatine is helpful to both ends. Research has shown that creatine supplement users have significantly less heat illnesses, dehydration, muscle tightness, and cramping compared with nonusers. Athletes supplementing creatine have fewer sports-related injuries, particularly when training in heat.[36] This could be due to creatine's hydrating effect as it draws water into the muscles. Patients with kidney disease and frequent muscle cramps who start supplementing creatine also typically report significant improvement.[37]

Creatine supplementation during prehabilitation has multiple potential benefits. When combined with resistance training,

---

[35] Joanna Willis et al., "Protein and Creatine Supplements and Misdiagnosis of Kidney Disease," *BMJ* 340 (2010): b5027, https://doi.org/10.1136/bmj.b5027.

[36] V. J. Dalbo et al., "Putting to Rest the Myth of Creatine Supplementation Leading to Muscle Cramps and Dehydration," *British Journal of Sports Medicine* 42, no. 7 (2008): 567–573, https://doi.org/10.1136/bjsm.2007.042473; Michael Greenwood et al., "Cramping and Injury Incidence in Collegiate Football Players Are Reduced by Creatine Supplementation," *Journal of Athletic Training* 38, no. 3 (September 2003): 216–219, https://www.ncbi.nlm.nih.gov/pmc/articles/PMC233174/pdf/attr_38_03_0216.pdf.

[37] Chiz-Tzung Chang et al., "Creatine Monohydrate Treatment Alleviates Muscle Cramps Associated with Haemodialysis," *Nephrology Dialysis Transplantation* 17, no. 11 (November 2002): 1978–1981, https://doi.org/10.1093/ndt/17.11.1978.

creatine allows for greater strength and muscle gains and less pain after exercise. Creatine alone has minimal effect on muscle growth without exercise, but it may lessen loss of muscle mass (atrophy) during short-term inactivity.[38] This is very important for recovery after a surgery or treatment because vigorous exercise usually isn't feasible during this phase. Losing as little muscle mass as possible is hugely important.

Creatine may also benefit individuals with metabolic disease. Metabolic dysfunction-associated steatotic liver disease (MASLD), previously called nonalcoholic fatty liver disease, is becoming much more common in people with central obesity and metabolic disease. The good news is that studies have shown improvements in MASLD with creatine supplementation.[39] Through similar mechanisms in the brain, creatine may have antidepressant effects in certain individuals, but it's important to note that individuals starting creatine are also typically increasing their fitness participation.[40] Exercise has well-documented psychiatric and metabolic benefits that could be affecting depression just as much as creatine usage.

Even so, creatine is an accessible, powerful, safe supplement with the potential to boost exercise and metabolic health. It plays a major role in prehab supplementation. Creatine's most common side effects are nausea, bloating, and diarrhea, but these typically resolve quickly.

---

38 Richard B. Kreider and Jeffery R. Stout, "Creatine in Health and Disease," *Nutrients* 13, no. 2 (2021): 9, 14, 447, https://doi.org/10.3390/nu13020447.

39 Rafael Deminice et al., "Creatine Supplementation as a Possible New Therapeutic Approach for Fatty Liver Disease: Early Findings," *Amino Acids* 48, no. 8 (2016): 1983–1991, https://doi.org/10.1007/s00726-016-2183-6.

40 Mauricio P. Cunha et al., "Creatine, Similarly to Ketamine, Affords Antidepressant-Like Effects in the Tail Suspension Test via Adenosine A1 and A2A Receptor Activation," *Purinergic Signalling* 11, no. 2 (2015): 215–227, https://doi.org/10.1007/s11302-015-9446-7.

Protein and Your Diet

High-protein diets are commonly recommended for individuals interested in weight loss. Some individuals find this makes them feel full longer and leads to lower total calorie consumption. The body's "energy cost" of processing protein is also higher than carbs and fats, meaning the overall calories available for storage will be less with a high-protein diet. This phenomenon is called the thermic effect of food.

The current recommended dietary allowance (RDA) for protein is 0.8 grams per kilogram (2.2 pounds) daily; this is roughly 60 grams of protein for an individual weighing 165 pounds.[41] This recommendation was not intended as an upper limit but instead is the amount of daily protein estimated to avoid breakdown of muscle tissue. That's a low bar to clear for the average individual, but it's also objectively inadequate for patients who require extra protein, such as individuals with cancer, in surgery recovery, or with above-average physical activity.

As we age, our bodies use protein less efficiently. To complicate matters, plant versus animal protein makes a difference. Some plant proteins are worse at meeting metabolic demands because the protein is bound to fiber or contains a lower concentration of important amino acids. This doesn't mean plant protein is bad, only that you should understand the source of protein when determining your requirements.

This all implies target protein intake should be *at least* 1.2 to 1.6 grams per kilogram of body weight (approximately 0.75 grams per pound).[42] For a 165 pound individual, that's roughly

---

41 Daniel A. Traylor et al., "Perspective: Protein Requirements and Optimal Intakes in Aging: Are We Ready to Recommend More Than the Recommended Daily Allowance?," *Advances in Nutrition* 9, no. 3 (May 2018): 171–182, https://doi.org/10.1093/advances/nmy003.

42 Stuart M. Phillips et al., "Protein 'Requirements' Beyond the RDA: Implications for Optimizing Health," *Applied Physiology, Nutrition, and Metabolism* 41, no. 5 (May 2016): 565–572, https://doi.org/10.1139/apnm-2015-0550.

112 grams of protein, or around 35 grams at each of three meals. Some research recommends intake as high as 2 grams per kilogram a day, especially in older adults or in individuals with significantly elevated protein requirements.[43] *Anabolic resistance* is the reduced sensitivity to stimulation of muscle-building pathways from the diet that leads to reduced muscle mass. Individuals could potentially overcome this by maximizing protein intake, particularly animal sources rich in the amino acids leucine, lysine, and methionine.[44]

Protein timing is a strategy to reverse the natural muscle breakdown that occurs while we sleep and immediately after exercise. For certain individuals new to exercise, eating protein within two hours of exercise maximizes the muscle-building benefits of resistance training. Just as muscle catabolism is muscle breakdown for energy/nutritional building blocks, anabolism builds muscles. Our goal is to promote as much anabolism as possible because bedrest following surgery can lead to rapid strength declines, muscle loss, and worsened anabolic resistance. This process can occur much faster in older adults.[45]

Animal and plant proteins rich in the amino acid leucine may have direct benefits for insulin sensitivity. Recall that type 2 diabetes mellitus (formally "adult onset") is the result of insu-

---

[43] Anne Marie Beck and Mette Holst, "Nutritional Requirements in Geriatrics," in *Interdisciplinary Nutritional Management and Care for Older Adults: An Evidence-Based Practical Guide for Nurses*, ed. Ólöf G. Geirsdóttir and Jack J. Bell (Springer, 2021), 19–30, https://doi.org/10.1007/978-3-030-63892-4_2.

[44] Donald K. Layman et al., "Defining Meal Requirements for Protein to Optimize Metabolic Roles of Amino Acids," *The American Journal of Clinical Nutrition* 101, no. 6 (June 2015): 1330S–1338S, https://doi.org/10.3945/ajcn.114.084053.

[45] Gianni Biolo et al., "Anabolic Resistance Assessed by Oral Stable Isotope Ingestion Following Bed Rest in Young and Older Adult Volunteers: Relationships with Changes in Muscle Mass," *Clinical Nutrition* 36, no. 5 (October 2017): 1420–1426, https://doi.org/10.1016/j.clnu.2016.09.019.

lin insensitivity. These indirectly support insulin sensitivity by increasing glucose uptake by muscle in the short and long terms.

A high-protein diet isn't necessarily a one-size-fits-all strategy. Patients with liver and chronic kidney disease have historically been advised to limit protein consumption. Regarding cirrhosis, (advanced liver disease) practitioners do this to minimize the risk of elevated ammonia, which is a byproduct of protein metabolism and can cause confusion, fatigue, and even coma. Alternatively, these patients are also at high risk of frailty, making them vulnerable to other serious complications, and high-protein diets are a critical tool in treating this. As research on the benefits of high-protein diets piles up, the evolving recommendation is for these individuals to gradually increase daily protein intake to 1.2 grams per kilogram of body weight.[46]

Many studies tying protein to a negative impact on kidney function have a few issues. First, study participants were more likely to have faster kidney function decline because of other illnesses, such as recent heart attacks, high blood pressure, and diabetes.[47] Second, the few recurring negative associations were typically between *animal* protein sources and kidney disease. People who eat more animal proteins than vegetable proteins (*not* as part of a muscle-building, health-focused diet) are also more likely to smoke, have high blood pressure and diabetes, and be less active. Third, high-processed meat-based proteins—i.e., fast food—are also higher in salt and sugar. In addition to fructose, animal proteins from meat increase uric acid levels, and individuals with chronic kidney disease have more difficulty

---

46 Javier Lizardi-Cervera et al., "Hepatic Encephalopathy: A Review," *Annals of Hepatology* 2, no. 3 (July–September 2003): 127, https://doi.org/10.1016/S1665-2681(19)32137-4.

47 B. L. Kasiske et al., "A Meta-Analysis of the Effects of Dietary Protein Restriction on the Rate of Decline in Renal Function," *American Journal of Kidney Diseases* 31, no. 6 (June 1998): 954–961, https://doi.org/10.1053/ajkd.1998.v31.pm9631839.

excreting uric acid from the body.[48] Increased uric acid can worsen kidney function, leading to excreting less uric acid into the urine.

Based on these samples, protein alone shouldn't be framed as *the* culprit for worsening kidney function.[49] In individuals with chronic kidney disease, maintaining muscle mass is associated with longer healthspan (improved function in late life) and lifespan. The easiest way to achieve this is through resistance training and adequate protein consumption. A high-protein diet alone during the duration of prehab is very unlikely to impact kidney function.

The individual without advanced kidney disease who consumes a high-protein diet while exercising, not smoking, and eating vegetables and less sugary fruits can find it effective for building muscle while losing weight.[50] A great way to further lessen concerns is to consume protein from lean meat, dairy, protein isolates like whey, and vegetables while limiting protein from red meat.

What we eat, especially during prehab, is important. When we eat and how often can be just as critical.

---

48 Hyon K. Choi et al., "Intake of Purine-Rich Foods, Protein, and Dairy Products and Relationship to Serum Levels of Uric Acid," *Arthritis & Rheumatism* 52, no. 1 (January 2005): 283–289, https://doi.org/10.1002/art.20761.

49 Gang-Jee Ko et al., "The Effects of High-Protein Diets on Kidney Health and Longevity," *Journal of the American Society of Nephrology* 31, no. 8 (August 2020): 1667–1679, https://doi.org/10.1681/ASN.2020010028.

50 Allon N. Friedman et al., "Comparative Effects of Low-Carbohydrate High-Protein Versus Low-Fat Diets on the Kidney," *Clinical Journal of the American Society of Nephrology* 7, no. 7 (July 2012): 1103–1111, https://doi.org/10.2215/CJN.11741111.

Fasting Strategies

Many are aware that building muscle and exercising can potentially reverse type 2 diabetes.[51] Far fewer know that medically supervised fasting may potentially accelerate this process.[52]

For clarification of terminology, intermittent fasting (IF) switches between fasting and feeding days on a regular meal time schedule. Time restricted feeding (TRF) is when eating is limited to a certain number of hours each day. In the latter programs, typical feeding windows range from six to twelve hours daily. Both IF and TRF promote a weekly caloric deficit, or burning more calories than you take in. Increasing the time in a fasted state means there are simply fewer available hours to consume calories.

IF strategies rely on planned "fasting days" where no food is eaten for at least twenty-four hours. These can be grouped together, such as five fed days followed by two fasting days, or an alternate-day fast (alternating fed days and fasting days). TRF plans are sometimes inaccurately referred to as IF. Common TRF regimens may call for sixteen fasting hours to eight fed hours or twenty fasting hours to four fed hours.

Most fasting literature suggests that the primary pathway for weight loss is simply the average caloric deficit. Fasting shouldn't be taken lightly, as it can have risks. Patients on insulin or insulin-related medications could experience low blood sugar

---

51 S. Lee et al., "Relationships Between Insulin Sensitivity, Skeletal Muscle Mass and Muscle Quality in Obese Adolescent Boys," *European Journal of Clinical Nutrition* 66, no. 12 (2012): 1366–1368, https://doi.org/10.1038/ejcn.2012.142; Ronald J. Sigal et al., "Effects of Aerobic Training, Resistance Training, or Both on Glycemic Control in Type 2 Diabetes: A Randomized Trial," *Annals of Internal Medicine* 147, no. 6 (2007): 357–369, https://doi.org/10.7326/0003-4819-147-6-200709180-00005.

52 Rainer Stange et al., "Therapeutic Fasting in Patients with Metabolic Syndrome and Impaired Insulin Resistance," *Research in Complementary Medicine* 20, no. 6 (2013): 421–426, https://doi.org/10.1159/000357875.

(and maybe some irritability, being "hangry"), and multiday fasting may trigger gout flares or gallstones.[53]

The *best* lifestyle improvement is one that the patient can maintain. Some patients may find it easier to maintain an average calorie deficit through TRF or IF with a personalized feeding window instead of a daily, across-the-board caloric deficit. Scheduling feeding hours or days when there's social pressure to eat, such as work engagements, celebrations, or family meals, can maintain a feeling of normalcy while still meeting nutritional goals. Maintain high protein intake while in caloric deficit to minimize lean mass loss, although a little decrease in muscle mass is unavoidable. Building muscle is a core pre-procedural goal, which is why protein intake remains so important. In other words, we want there to be as little muscle breakdown as possible during fasting stages.

There are other strategies for weight loss with supporting research that is varied and contradicting.[54] Diets like low-carb, ketogenic, and low-fat or "themed" diets like the Paleolithic and Mediterranean diets are often only effective for certain people. For example, some individuals feel significantly less hungry and have less desire to eat when eating a ketogenic diet, which allows them to maintain a caloric deficit.[55] Others just don't. Ultimately, weight loss comes down to total caloric deficit—using more cal-

---

[53] Stephanie Welton et al., "Intermittent Fasting and Weight Loss: Systematic Review," *Canadian Family Physician* 66, no. 2 (February 2020): 117–125, https://www.ncbi.nlm.nih.gov/pmc/articles/PMC7021351/; Izzah Vasim et al., "Intermittent Fasting and Metabolic Health," *Nutrients* 14, no. 3 (2022): 631, https://doi.org/10.3390/nu14030631; Yiren Wang and Ruilin Wu, "The Effect of Fasting on Human Metabolism and Psychological Health," *Disease Markers* 2022 (2022): 1–7, 5653739, https://doi.org/10.1155/2022/5653739.

[54] Ju Young Kim, "Optimal Diet Strategies for Weight Loss and Weight Loss Maintenance," *Journal of Obesity & Metabolic Syndrome* 30, no. 1 (2021): 20–31, https://doi.org/10.7570/jomes20065.

[55] A. A. Gibson et al., "Do Ketogenic Diets Really Suppress Appetite? A Systematic Review and Meta-Analysis," *Obesity Reviews* 16, no. 1 (2014): 71, https://doi.org/10.1111/obr.12230.

ories than you take in. In some cases, diet type *may* change your caloric needs somewhat, but in the end, it's still calorie balance that matters for weight loss.[56]

How the body uses those calories can be icing on the cake. High-protein foods require more energy to digest, while high-fiber foods are incompletely absorbed. Thus, meals high in fiber and structured around high-protein foods take longer to digest and may promote a longer full feeling.[57]

Medically Supervised Fasting

The goal of medically supervised fasting is to make the body more sensitized to insulin, meaning the person will require less outside insulin or insulin-related medication. The fasting portion follows a period of restricting carbs and remaining on a stable diabetic medication regimen.

We can use different mechanisms of diabetes medications to understand how fasting helps. An alternative to injecting insulin can be medications like glipizide that increase the pancreas's release of insulin. Other medications like metformin lower blood sugar by decreasing glucose production by the liver (gluconeogenesis) or by increasing excretion of glucose from the body in urine or stool, including SGLT2 inhibitors (empagliflozin and canagliflozin) and metformin again, respectively. Prolonged fasting essentially functions like the latter non-insulin medications. Since no calories are consumed during a fast, the body uses glycogen (broken down to glucose) in the liver and muscles for fuel. Once these reserves are depleted, the body has room

---

56 Kim, "Optimal Diet Strategies," 26–27.

57 Thomas L. Halton and Frank B. Hu, "The Effects of High Protein Diets on Thermogenesis, Satiety and Weight Loss: A Critical Review," *Journal of the American College of Nutrition* 23, no. 5 (2004): 373–385, https://doi.org/10.1080/07315724.2004.10719381.

available to efficiently store glucose the next time a person eats. All that to say, immediate and long-term insulin requirements could decrease with a fasting regimen because the body has an easier time storing sugar with all of that newly available space.

One report summarized three patient experiences with medically supervised fasts. These patients had been diagnosed with diabetes for ten, twenty, and twenty-five years. They all required insulin prior to fasting, and once the trial started, the patients fasted three days per week for seven to eleven months. All three were off insulin in the first month. One patient was weaned from insulin in only *five days*. These patients also reported feeling much better, with some reporting more energy.[58]

This study tracked patients working closely with a specialized team, and this close supervision could have had an impact on their results. This type of lifestyle change should never be attempted without very close supervision given the risk of volatile changes in blood sugar and electrolytes. But it's likely that the results came from a combination of exercise, low-carb dieting, *and* the fasting program. Fasting is a no-cost intervention that can halt the forward progress of diabetes and begin walking back insulin requirements.

As a side benefit, fasting could also serve as an "elimination diet" for patients with food intolerances. Easing into the fast with a stepwise elimination of certain food times (dairy, gluten, etc.) may help you finally determine which has been causing your bloating, diarrhea, or other symptoms.

The lifestyle interventions that make up this pillar of prehab are diverse and can be quite powerful. Many of them serve to

---

58 Suleiman Furmli et al., "Therapeutic Use of Intermittent Fasting for People with Type 2 Diabetes as an Alternative to Insulin," *BMJ Case Reports* 2018 (October 2018): bcr-2017-221854, https://doi.org/10.1136/bcr-2017-221854.

make the exercise pillar more effective, but most can still be effective on their own. They also serve to benefit the third and final pillar, which has everything to do with a patient's mind, brain, and sensory experiences.

THE NEUROPSYCHIATRIC PILLAR

At some point, you might have heard a phrase along the lines of "We exist in our heads." It's easy to overlook this pillar in favor of interventions that directly impact our bodies, but the neuropsychiatric side of things will always be extremely important. This especially hits home during prehabilitation, when there is almost always stress or anxiety leading up to a major surgery or treatment.

This pillar is a crucial early component of prehab, whether a patient has been diagnosed with cancer, requires bariatric surgery, is undergoing a hip replacement, or any other prehab scenario. One of the most fundamental pieces of all things neuropsychiatric boils down to how a person feels—their mood—as this affects every treatment that comes later.

Mood and Stress

The motivation for a prehabilitation program—whether it be elective joint replacement, bariatric surgery, cancer treatment, etc.—can have a big impact on a patient's mood. For instance, the journey through cancer treatment may be long and difficult, and the burden may be so heavy that psychiatric support is vital. Bariatric surgery may be similar due to the stress of surgery and recovery, as well as risk of new or worsening addiction. Patients pursuing elective joint replacements who are living with chronic pain may have developed maladaptive behaviors. Mood disorders can increase pain perception, and treating the former may lead to improvements in the latter.

For patients with obesity, this mood assessment and treatment is particularly relevant. The association between obesity and depression goes in both directions, with a stronger link in women.[59] Mood and appetite are linked, as are stigma and mood. Treating depression can improve a patient's willingness to pursue change, and eventual weight loss may improve depressive symptoms. Bariatric surgery is likely to improve depression and binge eating disorders, but it may increase the risk of new or recurring disorders like substance abuse, restrictive eating disorders, and thoughts of self-harm in some.

With mood therapies comes the very important and related topic of stress management.

Methods for reducing stress play an important role in prehab. Besides exercise and psychiatric consultation, massage therapy and saunas can be effective and worthwhile. There is mixed data when it comes to massage therapy promoting recovery after exercise, but it could potentially lead to decreased fatigue, improved perceived recovery, and decreased soreness or muscle tenderness.[60] Reductions in soreness and improved perceived recovery may encourage ongoing exercise. It could also lead to decreased inflammatory markers and cortisol levels—objective signs that stress has been reduced.

---

[59] Nattinee Jantaratnotai et al., "The Interface of Depression and Obesity," *Obesity Research & Clinical Practice* 11, no. 1 (January–February 2017): 1–10, https://doi.org/10.1016/j.orcp.2016.07.003.

[60] Pornratshanee Weerapong et al., "The Mechanisms of Massage and Effects on Performance, Muscle Recovery and Injury Prevention," *Sports Medicine* 35, no. 3 (2005): 235–256, https://doi.org/10.2165/00007256-200535030-00004.

Heat therapy has long been used for sore, tight muscles.[61] Sauna is an effective way to apply heat over the entire body. It promotes muscle relaxation after resistance training, and studies have shown it can improve muscle function across various activities.[62] Hot water immersion is a similar stress reduction method. Both promote a chain of internal events that regulate protective pathways against different stressors. When it comes to recovery after exercise and less bodily stress, heat can be your friend.

Addressing Stigma

Stigma is an unfortunate yet real part of the neuropsychiatric pillar. Historically, individuals with a new diagnosis of certain cancers associated with unhealthy behaviors or individuals with obesity experience feelings of stigma. Patients with lung cancer often possess the highest levels of psychological distress of all cancers, largely the result of stigma suggesting the patients' behaviors caused the illness.[63]

Shame can be associated with anxiety and depression, leading to worse survival and quality of life in patients with cancer, regardless of whether they even actually smoked.[64] Likewise,

---

61 Hamish McGorm et al., "Turning Up the Heat: An Evaluation of the Evidence for Heating to Promote Exercise Recovery, Muscle Rehabilitation and Adaptation," *Sports Medicine* 48, no. 6 (2018): 1311, https://doi.org/10.1007/s40279-018-0876-6.

62 McGorm et al., "Turning Up the Heat," 1311–1328; Masaki Iguchi and Richard K. Shields, "Prior Heat Stress Effects Fatigue Recovery of the Elbow Flexor Muscles," *Muscle & Nerve* 44, no. 1 (July 2011): 115–125, https://doi.org/10.1002/mus.22029.

63 Janine Cataldo et al., "Measuring Stigma in People with Lung Cancer: Psychometric Testing of the Cataldo Lung Cancer Stigma Scale," *Oncology Nursing Forum* 38, no. 1 (2011): E46–E54, https://doi.org/10.1188/11.ONF.E46-E54.

64 Cati G. Brown Johnson et al., "Lung Cancer Stigma, Anxiety, Depression, and Quality of Life," *Journal of Psychosocial Oncology* 32, no. 1 (2014): 59–73, https://doi.org/10.1080/07347332.2013.855963.

individuals with obesity have long been accused of exhibiting overindulgent behavior—the association still exists despite neurobiologic proof that obesity is a disease exacerbated by a modern environment of caloric abundance. Often, individuals with obesity have experienced judgment and ridicule. This even manifests as bariatric surgery being considered "the easy way out."[65]

Mitigating stigma begins with healthcare professionals communicating clearly, openly, and inclusively. There is no room or time for judgment when it comes to prehab, and behavior modifications that do less harm can be more effective than puritanical, all-or-nothing recommendations. For example, cutting out sugary drinks is a better starting point than ordering a patient to consume three daily meals of lean meat, egg whites, and water. Vaporizing (vaping) nicotine may be a better recommendation than demanding a patient with a pack-per-day smoking habit quit on the spot, though research is still conflicted on this. The ultimate goal is to guide a patient to the healthiest habits, but small improvements at a time can lead to big sustainable changes in the end.

Such radical changes won't happen overnight. Trying to force change is less sustainable than being understanding. We must meet the patient where they are.

Sleep Optimization

Sleep is an underappreciated piece of supporting better health. Nearly limitless data supports the idea that every person should

---

[65] Lenny R. Vartanian and Jasmine Fardouly, "Reducing the Stigma of Bariatric Surgery: Benefits of Providing Information About Necessary Lifestyle Changes," *Obesity* 22, no. 5 (May 2014): 1233, https://doi.org/10.1002/oby.20721.

get at least seven hours of uninterrupted sleep per night—and some of us require a little "extra."[66]

Sleep isn't simply wasted time with the brain turned off and the body on layaway. These hours are crucial repair time, clearing waste products in the brain, recycling damaged proteins in the body, and rebuilding muscle fibers damaged by exercise.[67] That's just the beginning; there are many other restorative functions happening while we sleep.

Sleep is crucial for recovery following exercise. Sleep deprivation impairs the body's ability to store glucose in muscles, which is necessary for exercise performance and controlling blood sugar. Poor sleep slows muscle recovery and makes individuals more prone to injury.

Do you ever feel hungrier after a poor night's sleep? This is because the "hunger hormone," ghrelin, and a stress hormone, cortisol, increase while the "satiety hormone," leptin, decreases.[68] These changes make people prone to eating larger portions of more processed foods like cookies, chocolate, and potato chips. Chronic lack of sleep is associated with higher BMI, which is likely caused by multiple effects working together. The hormonal fluctuations from sleep deprivation make individuals more likely to store consumed calories, while also reducing the amount of calories burned.

There are scenarios where patients are sleepier than normal

---

66 Susan T. Harbison et al., "Selection for Long and Short Sleep Duration in *Drosophila Melanogaster* Reveals the Complex Genetic Network Underlying Natural Variation in Sleep," PLOS Genetics 13, no. 12 (2017): 1–46, e1007098, https://doi.org/10.1371/journal.pgen.1007098.

67 Kenneth C. Vitale et al., "Sleep Hygiene for Optimizing Recovery in Athletes: Review and Recommendations," *International Journal of Sports Medicine* 40, no. 8 (2019): 536, https://doi.org/10.1055/a-0905-3103.

68 Chia-Lun Yang et al., "Increased Hunger, Food Cravings, Food Reward, and Portion Size Selection after Sleep Curtailment in Women Without Obesity," *Nutrients* 11, no. 3 (2019): 8–9, 663, https://doi.org/10.3390/nu11030663.

in the daytime despite getting enough sleep. This could be a symptom of obstructive sleep apnea (OSA) or another sleep disorder that makes sleep less effective for recovery. These disorders can contribute to weight gain and metabolic dysfunction.[69] What happens next can turn into a self-perpetuating cycle where poor sleep promotes weight gain, which further worsens sleep.

Sleep apnea is associated with more negative effects than simply less sleep time from frequent awakenings. Sleep apnea consists of periods of absent breathing (apnea) and decreased breathing volume (hypopnea). These periods lead to increased sympathetic nervous system activity, which raises blood pressure and wakes the person from sleep. Moderate or severe OSA is associated with higher stroke risk. Severe OSA is also associated with coronary artery disease, and severe episodes can provoke heart attacks and arrhythmias.[70] Repeat episodes can result in permanent damage to arteries connecting the heart and lungs. In other words, obstructive sleep apnea isn't to be taken lightly. Along with poor sleep, it can lead to serious cardiovascular and lung issues.

Pain Management

Chronic illnesses often come with chronic pain, especially those requiring major prehab-worthy interventions like joint replacement, spine surgery, and limb amputation. Addressing pain in a

---

[69] Alex Gileles-Hillel et al., "Biological Plausibility Linking Sleep Apnoea and Metabolic Dysfunction," *Nature Reviews Endocrinology* 12, no. 5 (2016): 290–298, https://doi.org/10.1038/nrendo.2016.22.

[70] Jerome A. Dempsey et al., "Pathophysiology of Sleep Apnea," *Physiological Reviews* 90, no. 1 (January 2010): 72–84, https://doi.org/10.1152/physrev.00043.2008.

multimodal prehab program is a great way to maximize engagement in the plan's other aspects.

Chronic pain has a tendency to worsen sleep quality and mood. Improving pain will usually improve these other areas as well as quality of life after surgery or treatment.

Addressing pain often begins with setting realistic goals because fully eliminating pain isn't always possible. Our goal is to achieve tolerable pain levels and help patients return to doing the activities that pain has prevented. It can take time to improve behaviors and thought processes when people have lived with years of chronic pain. In complex cases where pain is debilitating and consuming, medications paired with counseling from a pain psychologist or mental health professional can have the greatest effect.

Pain is an unpleasant sensory and emotional experience. There is research that education and counseling to help patients identify pain as a neurologic symptom can be helpful in reducing pain after their intervention. Essentially, this allows individuals to visualize how they've increased their pain perception. With this understanding, patients have an easier time giving their pain less power, so to speak. These studies showed improved satisfaction after surgery and, in some cases, lower postoperative pain.[71]

Achieving pain control during prehabilitation is crucial for multiple reasons. There is likely to be post-intervention pain from things like surgery, chemotherapy, or childbirth. The prehab window offers time to figure out which pain management techniques are most effective for an individual before the

---

[71] Amy Waller et al., "Preparatory Education for Cancer Patients Undergoing Surgery: A Systematic Review of Volume and Quality of Research Output over Time," *Patient Education and Counseling* 98, no. 12 (December 2015): 1540–1549, https://doi.org/10.1016/j.pec.2015.05.008.

expected temporary increase in pain. We're able to test benefits from different medications, and resilience to chronic pain can be established before adding post-treatment pain. All of these factors can improve treatment outcomes and quality of life as well as cut down on the need for opioids.

Exercise, lifestyle, and neuropsychiatric interventions form the pillars that make up the foundation of a great prehabilitation program. The next chapter dives into the testing and medications that round out prehabilitation before breaking off into specific plans for different types of treatment. Remember, anything is possible with a plan.

ACTION POINTS

- The concept of delaying treatment to allow for health optimization through prehabilitation is often the more prudent strategy, even when treating cancer, and it is becoming more widely accepted. There are few interventions that cannot accommodate a time window for prehab.
- A key to prehabilitation is minimizing the burden of participation. Grouping appointments into one day can improve patient participation and minimize discouragement. Some individuals may highly benefit from meal delivery in order to get proper nutritional benefits.
- Personalized exercise regimens based on preferences are best—the best exercise is what you enjoy doing. This may begin with prescreening for patients with known signs or symptoms of cardiopulmonary, metabolic, or renal disease. The ideal exercise regimen includes resistance and aerobic activities to maximize benefits within limited time.
- Alternative exercise methods like aquatic therapy and blood-flow restriction training can be useful when a patient

is unable to bear weight or other exercises are too uncomfortable.
- Nutritional "nudges" can be more effective than strict diet requirements. Start by eliminating sugar-sweetened beverages and increasing protein consumption. High-protein diets that are properly designed and gradually introduced can likely even be tolerated by patients with advanced liver or kidney disease, at least during the prehab period.
- Fasting strategies can reduce calorie consumption without requiring constant calorie restriction. Some may improve metabolic flexibility and increase insulin sensitivity.
- Treating pain, mood disorders, and sleep disturbances may improve quality of life and treatment outcomes and help other prehab interventions to become more effective.

CHAPTER 2

DIAGNOSTICS AND MEETING YOUR MEDS

I'M JUST GOING TO COME RIGHT OUT AND SAY IT: I *LOVE* DRUGS (obviously the kind that come in small, orange, professional-looking bottles). I love learning about ones we've had on the market since the 1950s. I love learning about the ones breezing their way through clinical trials because they're absolutely dunking on the current "standard of care." I can't name my favorite professional sports team, but I definitely have a favorite angiotensin II receptor blocker (telmisartan), favorite nerve pain medications, and a favorite sleep medication or two—and neither of them rhyme with "b-Ambien."

I think I can hear appalled gasps through the pages, screen, or speakers, for our audiobook listeners. But wait. I don't think you should take more drugs. I think you should be taking *less* drugs, and this starts with a thorough understanding of how these drugs work both on their target receptors and on off-target sites, creating side effects. Sometimes, these side effects can be useful when treating other issues, like prescribing a certain antidepressant because it also promotes sleepiness. Or choosing a different antidepressant because when paired with an opioid receptor blocker, it is a highly effective weight-loss medication. By obsessing over the fine print of these medications, we can potentially squeeze the greatest benefit out of a handful of high performers and, when we pair them with other health strategies, end up using less total medication overall.

Now, picture yourself or a loved one being wheeled down a hallway and into an MRI machine inside a sterile, white room. The discomfort doesn't stop there. A cage is placed on your face, and you're told to lie still for several hours while the machine collects a detailed image of your body.

This is the type of situation some people avoid at all costs—a complete lack of control while things they may not fully understand are happening. All the medical interventions in this book come with a list of tests and screenings, not all of them entirely pleasant. It's easy to feel powerless as you're being wheeled into an MRI machine, just as it can be stressful to have a team of doctors poke and prod at you with varying levels of communication and compassion.

The best way to approach this type of situation is to remember that there's a purpose behind each one of these tests, a method to the discomfort. Yes, it's not ideal, but with knowledge as to what's happening and why comes peace of mind. Our goal is to help make that peace of mind possible by explaining specific diagnostics and medications and why they're important.

There are few singular silver bullets in medicine. That's especially true when it comes to prehabilitation, where multiple pillars are required to best prepare a patient for treatment. The issues we're tackling are often complex, meaning prehab must match that complexity and treat a person physically, mentally, and emotionally. Overlooking one factor, just like overlooking one part of the body, can have unintended consequences.

This chapter details the most common screenings for specific interventions as well as the strategic use of medications and supplements that can make exercise easier and more effective, reduce pain, and improve your quality of sleep. There are so many options that figuring out what works best, or what even applies to your situation, might feel overwhelming. This chapter will break down which tests, medications, and supplements are most important for the different pillars of well-designed prehabilitation.

DIAGNOSTICS IN A NUTSHELL

Diagnostics are critical for spotting disorders and determining a proper plan of action. Specifically, these are tests and screenings that identify a disease, condition, or injury based on signs and symptoms. Preparation can make a huge difference—that's the main premise behind prehabilitation, after all—and knowing ahead of time what might be asked of you or what tests will be used can help a patient feel more in control.

Much of what follows will be geared toward people dealing with obesity and metabolic issues like diabetes. Not every test or screening will be relevant for patients with frailty, but we'll make that distinction when necessary.

WEIGHT AND ACTIVITY HISTORY

Outside of the standard medical and surgical history questions, the first prehab questions a medical professional might ask have to do with getting to know a patient's weight highs, lows, successes, and sticking points.

Medical professionals need to know a person's highest weight and whether that is now (when the person is preparing for prehab) or at a previous point in their life. Being down from the highest weight is a good thing, but your team needs to know if that was deliberate or caused by illness. Rapid or unintentional weight loss can especially come with a loss of muscle mass in the process, and if the weight loss was unintentional, it may signify some other unknown underlying issue. That might make a person worse off even though they look "healthier" on paper. Losing significant muscle can be an issue before surgery.

During cancer treatment, the goal is often weight *maintenance* because gain and loss both have potentially negative implications. Weight gain—unless it's due to gaining muscle mass—may worsen metabolic issues, while weight loss can push a person toward frailty and malnutrition.

What strategies a person has tried in the past to lose (or gain) weight are also key. What worked, and what didn't? Data gathered with this inquiry may increase the efficiency of your prehab program. The exact strategies may not stay the same, but this can shed light on which weight loss medications, caloric restriction strategies, and exercise programs are most effective.

A person's prehab plan will depend on their starting health/physical fitness level, medical history, and upcoming treatment. Again, preceding cancer treatment and organ transplants, for example, a patient's goal is to maintain weight while preferably changing their body composition through diet and resistance training, while weight loss during prehab is much more important for something like bariatric surgery or joint replacement (in patients with obesity). Part of this is learning about a patient's current diet, exercise preferences, past surgeries, and any over-the-counter or prescription medications. Supplements and seemingly benign things like Tylenol PM might not immediately come to mind, but they're also relevant.

If you have tried diets in the past, which did you find easiest to maintain? For example, ketogenic diets don't work for some because they find it extremely difficult to maintain the nearly zero carb requirement. Others prefer "going keto" because it best controls hunger.

The same strategy applies for exercise and figuring out which type you're most comfortable doing. Whether it's the treadmill, rowing, weights, or speed walking, there's a form of exercise for everyone. It doesn't matter as long as you can stick with it, and we'll fine-tune things from there. Familiarity is a big plus because it cuts down on needed instruction and limits the risk of injury—the path of least resistance, essentially. In prehab, getting hurt is a setback we can't afford because if you get hurt you can't be consistent. And with everything, consistency is key.

Don't be surprised if you're asked about a history of disordered eating. Many people don't consider their behaviors "disordered" until reflecting on an obsession over calorie counting or anything that becomes borderline pathologic and adds to anxiety. A big part of healthy eating is making it less obsessive and decreasing associated anxiety. For example, allowing yourself "cheat meals" can relieve some of the pressure, as long as it doesn't become a slippery slope to worsening self-control. Knowing if a person has a history of disordered eating is important for the psychological aspect but also for choosing the right medications.

Certain anti-obesity medications work especially well for people with eating disorders because they can affect the reward pathway signaling associated with binging. On the other hand, some medications are dangerous for people with bulimia because they carry a risk of seizures. That's why it's important for medical professionals to be aware of all disordered eating patterns. Do you binge eat after everyone goes to sleep? Have you felt shame after eating? Relevant parts of a patient's life might not seem relevant until examined objectively.

We'll also need to explore weight-related comorbidities (multiple conditions at once). This is about treating the patient "as a whole," but it also plays a role, unfortunately, in insurance coverage. Let's take a look at someone with diabetes and a BMI of thirty-two (on the low end of what's considered obesity). This person might qualify for newer medications that treat both obesity and diabetes in one. Now consider a person with a BMI of thirty-four without any other comorbidities. Even though they have a higher BMI, they may not be a candidate for a drug like semaglutide or tirzepatide (Wegovy and Zepbound) because they're deemed "too healthy." Analogous considerations can happen on the other end of the spectrum when it comes to treating frailty.

Obesity is often involved when we're talking about comorbidities. Obesity is broken into three groupings: class I, class II, and class III. Class III is what is sometimes referred to as "severe" or, previously, "morbid" obesity. Again, classification may play a role in what medications are most effective and what's covered by insurance. Obviously, a goal of prehab is for individuals to lose fat, even if they aren't losing weight. But we can't treat obesity properly and safely until we dive deeper into family history.

Knowing if a patient has a family history of certain types of cancers is potentially crucial. Semaglutide is an example of the new, injectable protein class of weight-loss medications. These drugs can be quite effective, but there is an uncertain (but presumed low) risk of them provoking one type of thyroid cancer. The recommendation at the time of this writing is not to prescribe these drugs to individuals with a history of *medullary* thyroid cancer or multiple endocrine neoplasia (MEN), with the latter being an inherited condition. Certain medications may also cause pancreatitis, which in some cases can be fatal. Overally, these types of history questions may seem oddly specific, but they're posed for good reasons.

Beyond patient and family history and comorbidities, your prehab team needs to take a closer look at your current activity level. Focusing only on "exercise" is too specific; certain activities that don't feel like exercise *actually* can burn meaningful calories or promote better health.

I've had patients who work at a daycare but don't have time for exercise. They chase kids around all day and end up easily getting 10,000 daily steps. While I'd love for them to add resistance training into their schedule, this current activity is far better than nothing. Childcare like this is meaningful activity—just like a baggage handler at the airport is far from sedentary. Quantifying a person's activity levels is about looking at their non-exercise activities as much as exercise.

Your team takes this into consideration before planning exercise recommendations. A person with plenty of aerobic activity in their day-to-day life might benefit more greatly from prioritizing resistance training. Someone who lifts heavy things for a living might be better off first adding some general aerobic conditioning.

Just as we overviewed in the last chapter, how we exercise is directly connected to our diet. If a patient tends to eat the same thing everyday, dietary questioning can be more simplistic. If his or her diet has a wide variety, it's important to get an idea of the extremes by asking more detailed questions. That being said, food recall surveys after the fact are often unreliable, so using an app or food journal to track daily meals is a great way to overcome human error.

The natural transition in the history sequence from food and exercise is sleep. The STOP-BANG and Epworth Sleepiness Scale are two popular sleep-related screening tests.[72] Checking these out ahead of time can prepare patients for questions they'll be asked, including the following:

- "How likely are you to fall asleep at red lights, in meetings, while watching TV, etc.?"
- "Do you snore loudly?"
- "Is your neck above sixteen inches around?"

These types of questions screen for sleep apnea and other sleep disorders. For instance, there is a fairly strong relationship between neck circumference greater than sixteen inches and sleep apnea. Sleep questions might not seem all that important, but they're part of peeling back the onion on details that may have an outsized impact on health.

EXAMS TO EXPECT

Again, knowing what to expect can ease some of the apprehension about visiting the doctor.

It's pretty safe to assume that any physical exam will begin with measuring your height and weight. These numbers, particularly weight, are useful to monitor trends over time, but they are also the inputs for calculating a person's body mass index (BMI). BMI is an easy, albeit imperfect, screening method to determine if a person is underweight, overweight, or in a healthy weight range.

---

[72] Mahesh Nagappa et al., "Validation of the STOP-Bang Questionnaire as a Screening Tool for Obstructive Sleep Apnea Among Different Populations: A Systematic Review and Meta-Analysis," *PLOS One* 10, no. 12 (2015): 1–21, e0143697, https://doi.org/10.1371/journal.pone.0143697.

There are exceptions, like if a person is muscular. They'll have a high BMI, but it might not necessarily be considered negative. Because BMI is a "quick and dirty" way to estimate body fat, we can measure waist circumference to make BMI a more accurate predictor of illness. If a patient's BMI is over twenty-five but they have a narrow waist circumference, that BMI number isn't necessarily indicative of metabolic illness. The reverse can be true. A person with a relatively low BMI but a larger waist circumference might not be as healthy as their BMI implies. BMI uses height and weight to guess body composition, but adding a waist measurement can make that number more accurate. Of course, higher body fat is associated with higher risk for metabolic illness.

The next measurement may be neck circumference. This has less to do with BMI and body fat and more to do with sleep apnea risk. As already mentioned, sleep apnea is more important than people might think because it leads to many other serious conditions. All else held equal, a neck circumference of sixteen inches or less is preferred, though the exact impact varies by height and sex.

Next, we have tools to better determine body composition. There are several ways to approach this, but the three most common methods are via DEXA, calipers, and bioelectric impedance.

Dual X-ray absorptiometry (DEXA) uses low levels of X-rays to measure bone density and different tissue balances like body fat and lean mass.[73] This scan is quick and painless. A CT scan or MRI is also effective for this purpose, but both of these are far

---

[73] David L. Kendler et al., "The Official Positions of the International Society for Clinical Densitometry: Indications of Use and Reporting of DXA for Body Composition," *Journal of Clinical Densitometry* 16, no. 4 (October–December 2013): 496–507, https://doi.org/10.1016/j.jocd.2013.08.020.

more expensive and time consuming, which makes DEXA often the preferred tool. Even less sophisticated, calipers are devices used to measure skinfold thickness at specific sites on the body. These measurements are converted into a body fat percentage using special algorithms. Calipers aren't the most accurate way to measure body composition, but they're relatively inexpensive and easy to use in the right hands.[74]

The final, and arguably most common, method to measure body composition is through bioelectric impedance. This is as easy as standing on a scale, only in this case the scale sends a painless amount of electricity into your body. The machine then measures the amount of electrical resistance to that current traveling through the body. A lot of resistance points to a higher amount of body fat. Lower resistance indicates more muscle because muscle contains water and electrolytes, which conduct electricity better. This estimates the fat-to-lean-mass balance. Home versions of this technology are available, but the equipment at a hospital or doctor's office will typically be much more accurate.

LAB TESTING AND BLOOD WORK

Lab tests are important for a number of reasons. Knowing how key metrics relate to different conditions can be useful for anyone beginning a prehab program. Fasting blood sugar and hemoglobin A1c (HbA1c) are crucial screening metrics for people at risk for diabetes. Measuring a person's lipids—cho-

---

[74] Jason R. Beam and David J. Szymanski, "Validity of 2 Skinfold Calipers in Estimating Percent Body Fat of College-Aged Men and Women," *Journal of Strength and Conditioning Research* 24, no. 12 (December 2010): 3448–3456, https://doi.org/10.1519/JSC.0b013e3181bde1fe.

lesterol and triglycerides, primarily—can indicate the potential for heart disease and other issues.

Doctors measure liver enzymes to help determine the health of a person's liver, with elevations suggesting fatty liver disease or other conditions. This can also help monitor progression or treatment of an existing disease. In the same vein, a basic metabolic panel (BMP) measures common electrolytes in the blood, along with a few other substances that include creatinine and glucose. One thyroid screening test (TSH level) is a good way to quickly screen for thyroid dysfunction. The thyroid regulates many functions throughout the body, chief among them being metabolism.

A complete blood count (CBC) is another important part of lab testing that comes into play when surgery or chronic disease are involved. It measures red blood cells, white blood cells, and platelets. Red blood cells carry oxygen throughout the body, and a CBC can determine if anemia—a lack of red blood cells or the hemoglobin component—is at play. Anemia is a concern prior to surgery, as all surgeries usually involve some (though usually low) amount of blood loss.

Finally, research is suggesting vitamin D may be more important than previously thought. Beyond bone health and immune support, abnormal vitamin D levels are associated with increased risk of some diseases, though, truly *causal* in few. If someone is vitamin D deficient, restoring them to a healthy level should be a top priority because treatment is simple and could make them feel better in general or help them respond better to certain treatments. There is ongoing debate if vitamin D *itself* is responsible for better health or if already healthy people have other behaviors that coincidentally raise their vitamin D levels, such as outdoor activities and a healthy diet.

Several lab tests are specifically tied to obesity and bariatric surgery. HOMA-IR is a relatively new test for insulin resistance.

Other obesity-associated conditions to potentially screen for include high cortisol (Cushing syndrome), polycystic ovary syndrome (PCOS) and hyperandrogenism in women, hypogonadism in men (popularized as "Low T"), elevated calcium score (atherosclerotic cardiovascular disease), low ankle brachial index (ABI, peripheral arterial disease), and any weight-related sleep disorders.

PCOS can be both a cause and effect of metabolic syndrome and infertility in women. Androgens are sex hormones like testosterone, and hyperandrogenism is a condition where a woman has high levels of androgens. Testing involves blood work and sometimes an ultrasound of the ovaries. Sticking with the androgen theme, hypogonadism in men is low testosterone. Insulin resistance can contribute to low testosterone, which can worsen body composition—storing more fat while losing muscle mass and bone density. Fixing these issues in the short term can spur a better response to exercise and nutritional plans.

A calcium score is a special CT scan of the heart that measures the cumulative effect of heart disease that has been chronically undertreated. This test isn't about calcium in your bones; it examines how much calcium has been deposited in the blood vessels of the heart. If that number is high relative to what's expected for age, it points to damage caused by smoking, high blood pressure, and high cholesterol.

We'll get into more detail on ABI testing in the amputation chapter, but this test checks the difference in blood pressure and blood flow at the level of the ankle versus the arm. Many conditions involving blood vessels are known as "length dependent"—the further from the heart, the more likely you are to see problems. Stiff blood vessels at the ankles are caused by the same risk factors as a high calcium score. This factors into a risk assessment of nonhealing wounds and amputations.

And once again, objective sleep testing falls into this category. Plethysmography is a component of the gold standard for detecting sleep apnea, polysomnography. This test evaluates breathing by measuring movement of the chest and abdominal wall. Since sleep apnea causes people to stop breathing for short periods while they sleep, plethysmography is a great tool for diagnosis. Then, polysomnography measures the effect on actual brain waves during sleep.

These are most of the potential tests a prehab candidate could undergo. Depending on the type of treatment or surgery an individual is preparing for and their past medical history, certain tests may be used while others are irrelevant. For instance, someone preparing for a lower leg amputation due to a nonhealing wound and peripheral vascular disease will probably also get a calcium score. Bad blood vessels in the leg suggest bad blood vessels around the heart, making the test highly relevant for estimating surgical risk. Other prehab patients might never have a calcium score. Again, it comes back to relevance, but having broad knowledge of what to expect can only be a net positive.

WHAT WE LEARN

Screening and testing ultimately exist to help your physician infer current issues or anticipate future issues.

High waist circumference often correlates with the likelihood of an enlarged liver. This is a sign of fatty liver disease, which increases a person's risk of cirrhosis or liver cancer, among other negative outcomes. A thorough physical exam could identify findings like acanthosis, or darkening skin in the armpits and skin folds, which is often a sign of insulin resistance (prediabetes or diabetes).

Xanthomas are small, yellowish bumps on the skin caused

by excess fats/cholesterol in the bloodstream. These can appear anywhere on the body but often occur around joints and tendons. Similarly, corneal arcus is when there's a white, blue, or gray crescent around the cornea of the eye, like a discolored ring. These are signs of high cholesterol.

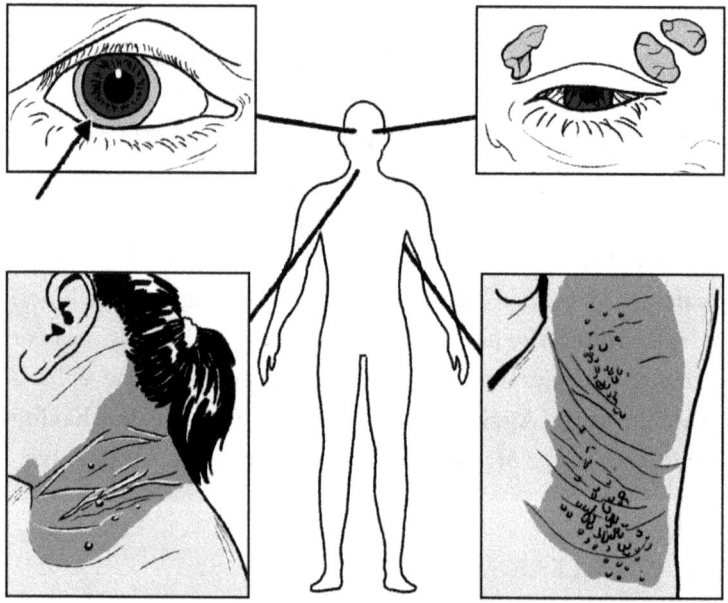

Sequelae of metabolic disease from top left counterclockwise: corneal arcus, xanthomas, and acanthosis nigricans of the axilla and neck

Distinct purple or pink stretch marks could be a sign of Cushing disease or syndrome. This implies that the body has excess cortisol or other corticosteroids in circulation. In Cushing disease, a tumor in the brain produces a hormone called ACTH that then tells the adrenal glands to produce cortisol. In Cushing *syndrome*, the body is either producing too much cortisol directly—a stress hormone—or a person is taking steroids for suppression of the immune system, and this can lead to quick loss of muscle mass and gaining fat around the abdomen, upper back, and face. Because of the muscle loss and fat gain, this is an unhealthy pattern that we'd prefer to avoid, but for some patients, steroid medications are necessary to control debilitating diseases like lupus (*systemic lupus erythematosus*) or rheumatoid arthritis or to prevent rejection after organ transplant.

Each of these can be potentially gleaned through screening and a physical examination. The final test that provides critical insights is an electrocardiogram (EKG). This is a safe and painless procedure where electrodes are placed on a patient's chest to record the heart's electrical activity. The electrodes don't produce electricity, so there's no risk of shock.

The most important purpose of an EKG is to quickly screen for any past issues or heart disease that weren't previously detected. For instance, an EKG can suggest something called cardiac remodeling. This is where the heart builds muscle or adapts due to things going on inside the body. A heart with more muscle in the left ventricle suggests that a person has had very high blood pressure for a long time. The heart wall thickens because it's trying to push against that resistance. After a while, this can lead to heart failure and other conditions.

An EKG can also identify old heart attacks or current electrolyte abnormalities. Some of these raise the risk of dangerous side effects from certain medications. The core theme of diagnostics is very true here: the more we know about a patient, in this case their heart, the better and more effectively we can treat them while avoiding complications. An EKG is pretty common across the board in prehab programs not only because it's important for prehab, but because surgeons and anesthesiologists often want EKG results in their preoperative workup.

In tandem with EKG testing, a stress test might also be used to try to provoke mild, relative ischemia to identify blood vessels that may already be narrowed. By further stressing the system, doctors can predict the likelihood of a future heart attack if this narrowing worsens. The benefit of a stress test prior to starting an exercise regimen is that it takes place in a controlled environment monitored by medical professionals, and it can detect areas at risk that aren't currently causing symptoms. The results can help your team tailor a safe but effective exercise program.

A CT or MRI of the brain is sometimes needed to look for different (usually benign) tumors that could cause hormone changes. These could affect adrenal gland production of cortisol, ovarian hormones like estrogen and progesterone, and testosterone from the testes. This latter scenario can cause infertility and low testosterone in men and women, affecting libido, mood, and energy levels.

That roughly covers the data-gathering portion of prehab preparation. Then comes the all-important question: what do we do with that information?

AN INTRODUCTION TO MEDICATIONS

You could think of medications in the prehab world in a similar way to screening and testing: they're tools helping us get where we're trying to go. They aren't miracle cures or silver bullets that wipe out disease, but when used along with a broader treatment strategy, medications can be highly effective. It can be empowering to know why a certain medicine is being prescribed beyond just hearing a catchy name and picking up the prescription at your local pharmacy. How specific medications work, why and when they're recommended, and how they contribute to wellness in the scope of prehabilitation are all important steps to getting back in the driver's seat.

EXERCISE PERFORMANCE AND RECOVERY MEDICATIONS

You may have noticed that in the United States, medications are heavily advertised. In fact, it's difficult *not* to notice. Perhaps no segment of the pharma world is as visible as drugs that can influence how we look. If you've turned on the television or browsed the internet recently, you may have come across the excitement around the newest medications used by patients and celebrities alike for diabetes and weight loss. Being that a pillar of prehab is largely about improving strength and physical recovery, it should come as no surprise that medications with the potential to improve physiology in these areas might play a role.

The following areas of research are designed to get *everyone* as excited about medications on the market (and in the pipeline) as your nerdy prehabilitation teammates, the author of this book proudly included.

AREAS OF RESEARCH—WHAT'S TAKING SO LONG?

The research pipeline for new medications or new indications/formulations of old medications is appropriately rigorous. However, due to this rigor, some medications may be abandoned during development despite some potential efficacy simply because the cost of continuing research exceeds the projected benefit to a manufacturer's financial bottom line. In other cases, a medication may proceed through regulatory approval for one condition but never "gain approval" for a different, completely reasonable use. Case in point, the medication gabapentin was originally approved for seizures and, now, nerve pain (neuropathy). Even though it has data supporting its significant benefit in improving deep sleep quality, it is unlikely to ever receive FDA approval for this purpose since gabapentin is currently available in generic formulations.[75] The money just isn't there to justify the investment in regulatory approval.

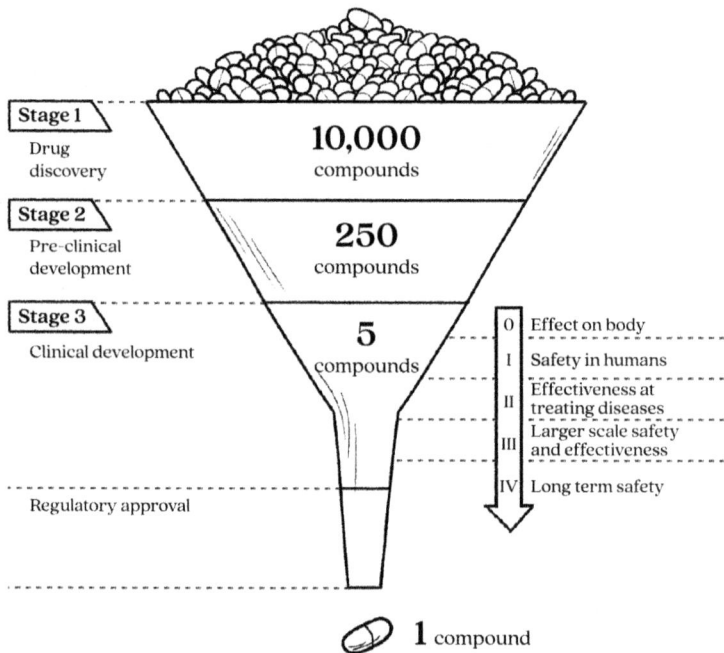

The rigorous process of identifying safe, effective medications and eliminating the rest

---

75 Yenan Shen et al., "Efficacy and Safety of Gabapentin in Improving Sleep Quality of Patients with Sensory Nervous System Diseases: A Meta-Analysis," *Alternative Therapies in Health and Medicine* 29, no. 5 (July/August 2023): 380–385, https://pubmed.ncbi.nlm.nih.gov/37235490/.

All of this is to say that some of the molecules listed below may never make it through the full regulatory process. Even so, I've included them here to introduce some of the relevant biochemistry that other medications may exploit for their side benefits. Also, understanding where researchers are currently looking provides reasons for optimism in the face of stubborn diseases that currently have few treatment options.

It's important to convey that just because we use a medication "off-label" does *not* mean it is necessarily a risky, Hail Mary, stab-in-the-dark attempt at experimenting carelessly in the face of limited evidence. In most cases, the medication likely has extensive research supporting its use for this off-label indication, and the benefits of using it in these cases may far exceed the risk of not having obtained formal FDA approval. Unfortunately, that approval may never come.

Myostatin Pathway Inhibitors

Ever see a photo of an extremely muscular dog, cow, or even child circulating the internet? This is usually when myostatin and other muscle-related proteins tend to gain attention.[76] Myostatin is a protein that limits the growth of muscles. In evolution, this served to minimize the number of calories an animal needed to survive; muscles require more calories to maintain than other bodily tissue.

Muscle eats up more calories, but it's also inversely related to metabolic disease. Because of this, researchers are successfully finding ways to break this evolutionary regulator. Or, in other

---

[76] Gina Kolata, "A Very Muscular Baby Offers Hope Against Diseases," *New York Times*, June 24, 2004, https://www.nytimes.com/2004/06/24/us/a-very-muscular-baby-offers-hope-against-diseases.html.

words, develop drugs that make it easier to build and retain muscle.

As anticipated, drugs that block the protein myostatin lead to increased muscle, decreased body fat, and improved blood sugar control.[77] This is an active area of research to treat multiple different conditions.

Exercise in a Pill

It's okay to get excited about this one, but let's keep things in perspective. Few of us would turn down something with all the benefits of exercise in pill form, but many medications have been touted as "exercise in a pill" over the years. Typically, this descriptor has simplified things to the point of untruth.

For now, peroxisome proliferator-activated receptor (PPAR) stimulators currently fall in the "too good to be true" category. PPAR stimulators (particularly PPAR delta subtypes) are arguably the closest science has come to truly achieving the claim of "exercise in a pill," particularly aerobic exercise. PPAR is a family of proteins that are applied to different functions in our cells, but mostly in the mitochondria, or the "powerhouse of the cell," as you've likely heard before. It should come as no surprise that the part of the cell that produces energy would be where this "exercise mimic" medication works.

This isn't really breakthrough technology. Doctors have been recommending other medications in this family for decades because they can have strong antidiabetic effects. However, research has shown that related drugs have the ability to stim-

---

[77] L. A. Consitt and B. C. Clark, "The Vicious Cycle of Myostatin Signaling in Sarcopenic Obesity: Myostatin Role in Skeletal Muscle Growth, Insulin Signaling and Implications for Clinical Trials," *The Journal of Frailty & Aging* 7, no. 1 (2018): 21–27, https://doi.org/10.14283/jfa.2017.33.

ulate our cells' power plants to increase the energy a person has for participating in exercise.[78] To generate this energy, mitochondria increase in number and become better at burning the "best" fuel source our bodies have—fat. This helps with exercise and could also promote brain and metabolic health (via fat loss).[79] Unfortunately, many drug candidates with the most potent activity have failed studies due to safety issues.

Selective Androgen Receptor Modulators

Anabolic steroids like testosterone have potential risks and side effects, so they're only recommended for individuals with abnormally low levels of this naturally occurring hormone. Researchers studying Selective Androgen Receptor Modulators (SARMs) ask the simple question, "Well, what if steroids didn't have those side effects?"

Essentially, that is the *intention* behind SARMs—to mirror the muscle-building, fat-burning, and insulin-sensitizing benefits of steroids like testosterone without negative consequences.[80] "Selective" in the name of these medications means that they selectively target those tissues—muscle and bone—while ideally avoiding activity in the liver, prostate, and heart.[81] When tied to prehab, this class of medications could theoreti-

---

78 Vihang A. Narkar et al., "AMPK and PPARδ Agonists Are Exercise Mimetics," *Cell* 134, no. 3 (2008): 405–415, https://doi.org/10.1016/j.cell.2008.06.051.

79 Anne Tailleux et al., "Roles of PPARs in NAFLD: Potential Therapeutic Targets," *Biochimica et Biophysica Acta (BBA)—Molecular and Cell Biology of Lipids* 1821, no. 5 (May 2012): 809–818, https://doi.org/10.1016/j.bbalip.2011.10.016.

80 Guadalupe Navarro et al., "The Role of Androgens in Metabolism, Obesity, and Diabetes in Males and Females," *Obesity* 23, no. 4 (April 2015): 713–719, https://doi.org/10.1002/oby.21033.

81 Varun S. Venkatesh et al., "The Role of the Androgen Receptor in the Pathogenesis of Obesity and Its Utility as a Target for Obesity Treatments," *Obesity Reviews* 23, no. 6 (June 2022): 1–21, e13429, https://doi.org/10.1111/obr.13429.

cally prevent muscle wasting, which often comes with inactivity before or after treatment. Anything that can prevent loss of muscle mass should be seen as a positive and may one day be on the table.

SARMs are not currently used in a clinical setting, although that could change in the future. Theoretically, they could be used while treating prostate cancer because they indirectly lower testosterone levels while still keeping the testosterone effect in parts of the body where it matters. This kind of use needs to be pursued going forward. To be clear, any currently "available" SARMs are unregulated, unapproved, and potentially dangerous.

SARMs are also relevant because they lead into a discussion of two important treatment types when it comes to exercise and recovery: hormone replacement therapy and testosterone replacement therapy.

Hormone Replacement Therapy

Throughout the 1980s and 1990s, physicians commonly prescribed hormone replacement therapy (HRT) for women suffering from symptoms of menopause. The logic was simple: replacing estrogen and progesterone would help relieve symptoms of hot *flashes*, fatigue, and sleep disturbance, among others. Then an imperfectly designed study came out suggesting that HRT may dramatically raise the risk of breast cancer. However, to simplify a long revision process, this risk number was corrected and contextualized until it was no longer statistically significant for most individuals.

The stigma around HRT still lingers, and many prescribers don't feel comfortable with the treatment due to lack of experience and safety concerns. But while the symptoms can be debilitating, HRT may offer distinct impressive longevity and quality of life benefits. It has been associated with lower risk of Alzheimer's disease and colon cancer and improved bone density.[82] HRT does come with some risks—potential for blood clots and gallstones—but the benefits are enough for many suffering women that it's returning to mainstream use. This conversation is long, nuanced, and definitely not "one size fits all."

Testosterone Replacement Therapy

The major sticking point with testosterone replacement therapy (TRT) was whether it would raise the risk of heart attacks. Overdoing TRT in a major way raises the liver's production of cholesterol, which could contribute to a heart-related event at some point. But that has nothing to do with TRT for the purposes of treating objectively low testosterone. Using TRT to bring people back to normal testosterone levels has many subjective benefits on wellness, and emerging data confirms no worsening of cardiovascular disease when restoring normal levels.[83]

Testosterone, as mentioned previously, is a hormone in both biologically male and female individuals that has many health benefits, including building muscle, burning fat, and indirectly supporting bone density through its muscle-building properties. Other prehabilitation-related benefits are increased energy for physical activity and faster recovery from exercise. When levels

---

[82] Noel S. Weiss et al., "Decreased Risk of Fractures of the Hip and Lower Forearm with Postmenopausal Use of Estrogen," *New England Journal of Medicine* 303, no. 21 (1980): 1195–1198, https://doi.org/10.1056/NEJM198011203032102.

[83] Vikash Jaiswal et al., "Association Between Testosterone Replacement Therapy and Cardiovascular Outcomes: A Meta-Analysis of 30 Randomized Controlled Trials," *Progress in Cardiovascular Diseases* 85 (July–August 2024): 45–53, https://doi.org/10.1016/j.pcad.2024.04.001.

are unnaturally low and a patient has symptoms that match this deficiency, prescribers should feel comfortable recommending TRT to treat symptoms and return levels to normal.

It's common for individuals with chronic disease to have low testosterone. This is worth fixing before starting a program aimed at building muscle and losing fat. Normal testosterone levels are essential to both of these goals, and postmenopausal women can even use very low doses of testosterone at times since menopause lowers testosterone in women. Researchers continue to study the long-term benefits of TRT, but current consensus is there are limited added risks and potentially significant benefits for health and wellness.[84] This is only for using TRT to reach normal testosterone levels. Using TRT to go above normal levels in men and women can raise cholesterol and cause acne, hair loss, voice changes (in women), and other "male-like" characteristics.

LIFESTYLE MEDICATIONS AND SUPPLEMENTS

Just as promoting a person's ability to exercise and recover is a major component of prehabilitation, so is using medications and supplements to promote a healthier lifestyle.

Gut Peptide Hormone

A handful of all-star weight-loss drugs currently on the market work by mimicking hormones released by different digestive organs. The copycatted hormones are glucagon-like peptide-1 (GLP-1), glucose-dependent insulinotropic peptide (GIP), and

---

[84] Giovanni Corona et al., "Testosterone and Cardiovascular Risk: Meta-Analysis of Interventional Studies," *Journal of Sexual Medicine* 15, no. 6 (June 2018): 820–838, https://doi.org/10.1016/j.jsxm.2018.04.641.

for weight-loss and fatty liver benefits, glucagon. It might be fair to say these medications are taking the medical world by storm as of the initial writing of this reference.

Semaglutide and tirzepatide are antidiabetic and anti-obesity medications. They have several non-weight/diabetes benefits as well, including protecting other organs from the negative effects of high blood pressure, lowering inflammation, and promoting brain health.[85]

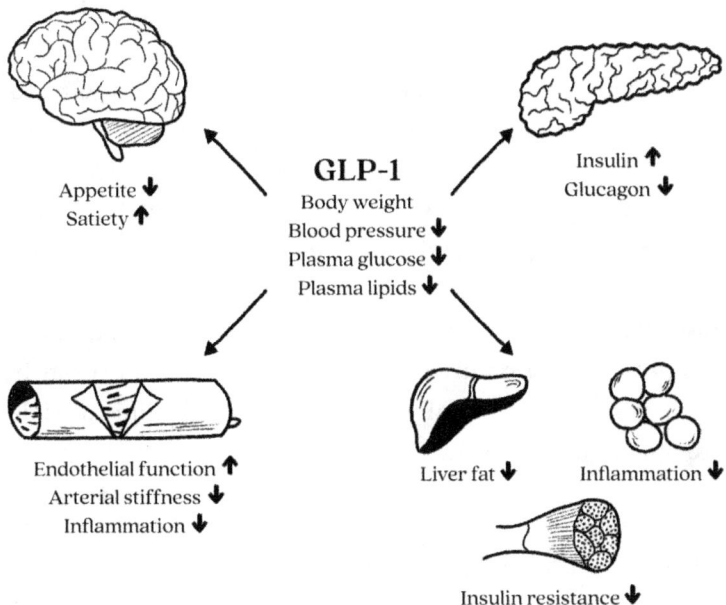

Known mechanisms by which GLP-1 receptor agonist medications improve weight and health

---

85 Søren L Kristensen et al., "Cardiovascular, Mortality, and Kidney Outcomes with GLP-1 Receptor Agonists in Patients with Type 2 Diabetes: A Systematic Review and Meta-Analysis of Cardiovascular Outcome Trials," *Lancet Diabetes & Endocrinology* 7, no. 10 (October 2019): 776–785, https://doi.org/10.1016/S2213-8587(19)30249-9; Isidro Salcedo et al., "Neuroprotective and Neurotrophic Actions of Glucagon-Like Peptide-1: An Emerging Opportunity to Treat Neurodegenerative and Cerebrovascular Disorders," *British Journal of Pharmacology* 166, no. 5 (July 2012): 1586–1599, https://doi.org/10.1111/j.1476-5381.2012.01971.x.

That doesn't mean these medications don't come with potential downsides. There are few "free lunches" (GI pun definitely intended) in medicine. Side effects include abdominal pain, nausea, vomiting, constipation, diarrhea, and even some anecdotal reports of "Ozempic face," or facial skin that sags and ages. The latter is likely due to rapid fat loss in the face that, over time, makes the user appear older, which can actually occur with *any* means of rapid weight loss.

The weight loss triggered by these medications is also a cause for concern. Yes, loss of fat mass can occur, but so can loss of muscle mass and bone density. There's no way around this; anything *that* effective at weight loss is going to make you lose muscle mass too. Trade-offs are a part of life. That doesn't mean these drugs need to be avoided. For some patients, the benefits—weight loss and improved diabetes, in particular—profoundly outweigh the negatives. In the future, other treatments like SARMs, myostatin inhibitors, and TRT could theoretically protect muscle mass and even promote muscle gain while taking these drugs. Presently, this has not been formally evaluated; though clinical trials are ongoing.

Two Old Dogs with New Tricks

Remember in the mid-1990s when the world's best basketball player and face of the NBA quit the sport that had made him millions? Michael Jordan left basketball in the fall of 1993 to pursue his other dream: baseball. He signed a minor league contract with the Chicago White Sox after not having played the sport since his senior year of high school. Essentially, he got signed sight unseen without a horde of talent scouts and front office people obsessing over film and analytics. His work ethic and athleticism from a different sport made for a comfortable understanding of drawbacks—his overly competitive nature, at times—and what he brought to the team...also his highly competitive nature. The White Sox were confident that Michael Jordan's skill set could be applied in a different way and knew about any shortcomings with which they'd potentially have to contend. His athletics journey is an excellent parallel to what we frequently see with reusing some medications today.

The beauty of new findings for old medications is that researchers can mix and match medications with long track records of safety for impressive new purposes. As a great example, to create the brand-name drug Contrave, pharmaceutical companies combined an antidepressant (bupropion) and a medication for alcohol and opioid addiction (naltrexone). Contrave serves an entirely new purpose as a prescription anti-obesity medication (weight loss drug).

Both individual medications had been on the market for decades, making prescribers extremely confident when it comes to their uses and safety. Bupropion is an effective antidepressant without the more common sexual and weight-promoting side effects of typical antidepressants. It also binds to nicotine receptors in the brain, making it helpful for people who are trying to stop smoking. Naltrexone has benefits in treating alcohol and opioid addiction, but new research shows potential anti-inflammatory benefits (at low doses) that may reduce chronic pain and even symptoms of multiple sclerosis.

Combining these drugs is where weight loss comes into play. The hypothalamus regulates appetite, and the combination (Contrave) can reduce some of the rewarding aspects of food that cause loss of control eating behaviors.[86] This effect leads to weight loss.[87]

The other drug combination worth discussing is phentermine and topiramate. Like the above example, these medications separately have long track records. Phentermine has been used for weight loss throughout its entire existence. It's structurally similar to amphetamines but doesn't invite misuse because it has limited impact on dopamine activity in the brain. However, it carries potential side effects like fast heart rate, high blood pressure, and anxiety. Phentermine is mostly an appetite suppressant but may promote a small amount of fat burning (*lipolysis*).

Topiramate was originally approved as an anti-seizure medication in the 1990s. Two decades later, it was approved for weight loss in combination with phentermine. The combination produces much more weight loss than either medication alone.

Orlistat

Orlistat is another weight-loss medication. It functions by blocking the enzyme that breaks down fat in our diets. Without this enzyme, fat travels through the stomach and intestines unabsorbed, which also means it carries a laxative effect. Simply put, orlistat keeps your body from absorbing fat.

The downside is that some vitamins can only be absorbed with fat. Individuals on orlistat may become deficient in these

---

[86] Andres Acosta et al., "Selection of Antiobesity Medications Based on Phenotypes Enhances Weight Loss: A Pragmatic Trial in an Obesity Clinic," *Obesity* 29, no. 4 (April 2021): 662–671, https://doi.org/10.1002/oby.23120.

[87] Tehane Ornellas and Benjamin Chavez, "Naltrexone SR/Bupropion SR (Contrave): A New Approach to Weight Loss in Obese Adults," *Pharmacy & Therapeutics* 36, no. 5 (May 2011): 255–262, https://pubmed.ncbi.nlm.nih.gov/21785538/.

vitamins. The drug may also affect the absorption of other medications. Finally, for many it only promotes modest weight loss—five pounds, according to some studies.[88] However, the response can be widely variable.

Based on limited effectiveness and the fact that it messes with absorption of other medications, orlistat is only prescribed for distinct situations. For individuals sensitive to stimulants who aren't on many medications and need only a "gentle" reminder (gas/diarrhea) to stay adherent to a diet, it may have benefit. For others, this is likely going to be a medication of last resort. We shouldn't completely discard this tool from the toolkit but understand its limitations.

OFF-LABEL INSIGHTS

Several medications exist that offer promising mechanisms for weight loss but aren't yet approved for weight loss at this time. They're worth discussing because (1) this could change in the future as more studies and reliable data come to light and (2) the unique mechanisms could be copycatted in the future to create even more effective medications with the sole purpose of weight loss.

Sodium Glucose Cotransporter 2 (SGLT2) Inhibitors

Think of SGLT2 inhibitors as an orlistat for diabetes, only more effective at reaching health-promoting goals. They cause the kidney to no longer reabsorb sugar when it's filtering blood,

---

[88] Amirhossein Sahebkar et al., "Effect of Orlistat on Plasma Lipids and Body Weight: A Systematic Review and Meta-Analysis of 33 Randomized Controlled Trials," *Pharmacological Research* 122 (August 2017): 53–65, https://doi.org/10.1016/j.phrs.2017.05.022.

allowing excess sugar to pass from the body in urine. A common negative side effect is urinary tract infections because sugar-rich urine is a favorable environment for growing bacteria and yeast. This attracts both bacterial and fungal infections and could even lead to a rare, but serious condition called Fournier's gangrene, "flesh eating" infection of the groin area. SGLT2 inhibitors' mechanism of action also "created" (really just increased the prevalence) of a previously rare and serious condition called euglycemic ("normal" blood sugar) diabetic ketoacidosis.

The really useful thing about SGLT2 inhibitors is that they have several other long-term benefits beyond simply controlling blood sugar levels. Research discovered that SGLT-2 inhibitors can offer protection to organs from accelerated aging of blood vessels and can even slow the progression of heart failure. People taking these drugs have fewer strokes and heart attacks and reversal of heart failure effects.[89] SGLT2 inhibitors also can protect the kidneys and are now being studied for longevity purposes.

While all that is great, there's a small caveat—these benefits offered by SGLT2 inhibitors are similar to many offered by GLP-1 receptor agonists (RA). Only, GLP-1 RAs can promote substantially more weight loss than SGLT2 inhibitors at their maximum dose. That means this class of drugs isn't the most effective out there at helping people lose weight, although they typically have fewer side effects and don't have to be injected like most GLP-1s. As such, SGLT2 inhibitors aren't great drugs for weight loss but can be excellent candidates to buddy up with other medications.

---

[89] Milton Packer, "SGLT2 Inhibitors: Role in Protective Reprogramming of Cardiac Nutrient Transport and Metabolism," *Nature Reviews Cardiology* 20, no. 7 (2023): 443–462, https://doi.org/10.1038/s41569-022-00824-4.

Mirabegron (and Other Beta-3 Adrenergic Receptor Agonists)

Mirabegron is a medication that calms the muscles of an overactive bladder. This medication is a perfect example of killing two birds with one stone. For metabolic health, it works by binding to the same receptors on fat cells, stimulates mitochondrial production, and increases lipolysis (burning fat). This promotes improvements in related metabolic processes like high LDL cholesterol and blood sugar levels.[90]

Like SGLT2 inhibitors, beta-3 agonists offer multiple benefits, but these won't be the main driver of weight loss. The weight loss it promotes isn't very pronounced, and taking too much can cause negative side effects like high blood pressure and fast heart rate.[91] Mirabegron alone isn't enough to lose serious amounts of weight, but it can help while also treating bladder issues. Research is ongoing for using related medications for metabolic purposes. Presently, however, these medications have not been approved for purposes outside of bladder overactivity.

Metformin

Metformin is another drug that has been used for decades to control blood sugar. Popular since the 1950s, few drugs have been taken by as many people over the years. It's also one of the

---

[90] Alana E. O'Mara et al., "Chronic Mirabegron Treatment Increases Human Brown Fat, HDL Cholesterol, and Insulin Sensitivity," *Journal of Clinical Investigation* 130, no. 5 (May 2020): 2209–2219, https://doi.org/10.1172/JCI131126.

[91] Rebecca K. C. Loh et al., "Acute Metabolic and Cardiovascular Effects of Mirabegron in Healthy Individuals," *Diabetes, Obesity and Metabolism* 21, no. 2 (February 2019): 276–284, https://doi.org/10.1111/dom.13516.

rare medications that still carries some weight when stacked up against newer drugs.

Similar to those new drugs, metformin can control blood sugar with minimal risk of hypoglycemia (dangerously low blood sugar) when used alone. It may also offer other benefits to organs in the body and promote weight loss. Metformin works by decreasing the total amount of sugar the body absorbs and produces itself. One downside is that it can cause nausea and diarrhea when starting the medication or increasing dosage. This usually doesn't last, but metformin also heightens the potential for acidic blood (acidosis) in individuals with liver or kidney disease. Finally, and most concerning for our purposes, it may reduce the beneficial response to exercise.[92] Metformin could be like putting your foot on the break in terms of exercise benefits. This is a major part of prehab, meaning that metformin isn't always the best option, depending on an individual's unique situation.

NEUROPSYCHOLOGY, SLEEP, AND PAIN MEDICATIONS

I can't overstate how important, yet overlooked, sleep is for self care. Poor quality or quantity of sleep is associated with disruption of hormones that control appetite and fat storage and even sex hormones. On top of that, messing up those hormones can worsen higher blood pressure and diabetes.

Sleep deprivation is rarely deliberate—often it's due to excessive workloads or insomnia related to stress. With these

---

92 Adam R. Konopka et al., "Metformin Inhibits Mitochondrial Adaptations to Aerobic Exercise Training in Older Adults," *Aging Cell* 18, no. 1 (February 2019): 1–12, e12880, https://doi.org/10.1111/acel.12880.

issues related to a mind that just won't calm down, many individuals reach for over-the-counter medications (Nyquil, Benadryl, or Tylenol PM), prescription sleep drugs (Ambien or Lunesta), or older medications like Valium, Xanax, and Ativan. These medications might seem like a quick fix, but the problem is they don't really promote *physiological* sleep. They kind of just turn everything off in most cases. That isn't helpful or healthy.

When studying the brain waves of a sleeping person who took one of these sleep medications, tests often show blunting of rapid eye movement (REM) sleep—a stage crucial for emotional wellness. Other medications affect deep sleep, which may result in impaired immune system functioning, leading to frequent illnesses and potentially higher cancer rates.

When given the choice, one potentially better prescription medication for sleep is trazodone, which was originally developed as an antidepressant. Trazodone was limited as an antidepressant because its main side effect was sleepiness. Studying sleeping individuals on trazodone has shown that they maintain normal "architecture," or their sleep is objectively normal. Another drug called mirtazapine (Remeron) has similar activity but can also relieve nausea and potentially stimulate appetite. This is a potential side benefit for someone with frailty or difficulty maintaining their weight due to chronic nausea. Both medications are not without side effects, but these are often (although not always) minor.

Certain supplements also aid sleep in a safe and effective way. Magnesium glycinate and magnesium L-threonate cross the blood-brain barrier and bind to GABA and NMDA receptors. Essentially, they use similar pathways as sleep drugs but are gentler and don't mess with REM sleep or your memory. The amino acid glycine also has the potential to improve sleep quality, as does the supplement ashwagandha.[93] Ashwagandha has been popular in Eastern medicine for a long time, and it has similar sedative effects to valerian root (another effective "natural" sleep aid).

The main problem with supplements is that meaningfully improving sleep requires a certain amount, and many over-the-counter supplements simply don't have a high enough concentration, aren't well absorbed, or don't contain what's listed on the label. These supplements can work, but only if you take a high enough dose. Otherwise, they may not have much effect over a placebo.

It's worth mentioning melatonin as a supplement, given its popularity. Melatonin is a hormone our brains naturally produce to control the sleep cycle. This natural release steadily decreases the level of arousal as the sun sets. The problem with this is that our lives are so filled with artificial light and screens that we become stimulated at night and less melatonin gets released. Avoiding blue light in the evening and wearing blue light-blocking glasses is one effective remedy. While melatonin supplements can be helpful, addressing the root cause is likely a better long-term solution.

All that is to say that quality sleep is critically important, particularly in prehabilitation, where there is so much emphasis on improving exercise and lifestyle. The good news is that when it comes to neuropsychology, sleep, and pain, there are numerous medications and treatments that may help. Improvement in this pillar will not only help the other two pillars but can provide

---

[93] Nobuhiro Kawai et al., "The Sleep-Promoting and Hypothermic Effects of Glycine Are Mediated by NMDA Receptors in the Suprachiasmatic Nucleus," *Neuropsychopharmacology* 40, no. 6 (May 2015): 1405–1416, https://doi.org/10.1038/npp.2014.326; Kae Ling Cheah et al., "Effect of Ashwagandha (*Withania Somnifera*) Extract on Sleep: A Systematic Review and Meta-Analysis," *PLOS One* 16, no. 9 (2021): 1–22, e0257843, https://doi.org/10.1371/journal.pone.0257843.

prehab participants a better quality of life and improved emotional state.

Nerve Pain and Antidepressants

The prominent class of newest antidepressants is the serotonin-norepinephrine reuptake inhibitors (SNRIs). Like the name suggests, they prevent those two chemicals—which impact our emotions, well-being, and happiness—from being inactivated. This leads to downstream effects on brain inflammation and neurologic stress response. In addition, these drugs have also found wide acceptance for their secondary benefit of pain reduction, particularly nerve pain. It stands to reason that because SNRIs improve pain in patients *without* depression, they are modulating some of the activity in our pain sensing pathway. They can suppress ascending pain signals—the signal traveling from nerves to the spinal cord and then the brain.

Chronic pain and depression/anxiety commonly occur together, which makes SNRIs particularly effective at breaking this pain cycle. Consider this scenario of the common vicious cycle of chronic pain:

You hurt your back lifting something. You "take it easy" and stop going to the gym for a week to let the injury rest. At the end of this sedentary week, your back still aches, bringing with it nagging worry—how long will this last? "Maybe I should go to the gym," you think, and you do your typical workout but stop halfway because of a jolt of lower back pain. Resting forever isn't an option, and there's work to consider. You return to your job and find that getting through the day is exhausting. A cloud of pain looms, darkening your mood and limiting participation in activities you used to enjoy. Everyone knows someone who has a chronically "bad back." It's natural to think, "Will this be me? I'm too young for that, but I can barely even walk upright some days."

This cycle of inactivity to avoid aggravating the injury, isolation, depression, weight gain, and more pain is often difficult to break once it gains momentum. The brain actually rewires to give this pain sensation and its association with certain movements more cerebral real estate. In other words, the more pain you sense/focus on, the more your brain looks for it, even in areas without tissue damage.

This is another reason antidepressants can be very effective pain medications. These medications attack part of the biochemistry of pain, but they also affect the mood (perceptual) component of pain. A better mood and less anxiety quiet the nagging voice telling the pain sufferer, "It's best to take it easy; you'd hate to risk making things worse." A better mood and more energy help a person dealing with pain to move their body and remind their brain that basic movements aren't going to hurt them. On top of that, better mood and sleep make it easier to choose healthier foods that stop weight gain, facilitate weight loss, lower inflammation, and break the chronic pain cycle.

SNRIs and the other two major classes of antidepressants, selective serotonin reuptake inhibitors (SSRIs) and tricyclic antidepressants (TCAs), are not all created equal. Some are relatively better for mood than pain, while others offer greater relief for common depression symptoms like insomnia and anxiety. Consulting with an informed medical professional makes it easier to find medications tailored to your unique symptoms. If pain is the main symptom, this strategy helps find the best option for pain relief with the fewest side effects. Physicians will also consider how medications interact with common prehab-related conditions like heart arrhythmias and electrolyte imbalances, among others.

Examples of common medications in each class:

- SNRIs: Venlafaxine (Effexor), desvenlafaxine (Pristiq, Khedezla), duloxetine (Cymbalta)
- SSRIs: Fluoxetine (Prozac), paroxetine (Paxil), sertraline (Zoloft), citalopram (Lexapro), escitalopram (Celexa)
- TCAs: Doxepin (Silenor), nortriptyline (Pamelor), amitriptyline (Elavil)

Seizure Medications

Similar to using antidepressants for nerve pain, medications originally developed for controlling seizures may be effective in treating nerve pain. Seizure drugs work by decreasing nerve cell activity. As neuropathic (nerve) pain could be caused by nerve injury or overactivity, these drugs are effective in treating various causes of pain like neuropathy, phantom limb pain, and neuromas.

Commonly used medications like gabapentin (Neurontin) and pregabalin (Lyrica) are widely prescribed yet rarely used as antiseizure medications.[94] These drugs are typically well tolerated and can complement other medications like SNRIs, making them early choices for nerve pain.[95] Side effects are generally mild and include dizziness, brain fog, and leg swelling, but these can cause injury if you're unprepared. They may also worsen side effects of other medications, such as sleepiness and even weight gain.

---

[94] Nathan J. Pauly et al., "Trends in Gabapentin Prescribing in a Commercially Insured U.S. Adult Population, 2009–2016," *Journal of Managed Care and Specialty Pharmacy* 26, no. 3 (2020): 246–252, https://doi.org/10.18553/jmcp.2020.26.3.246.

[95] Philip J. Wiffen et al., "Carbamazepine for Chronic Neuropathic Pain and Fibromyalgia in Adults," *Cochrane Database of Systematic Reviews* 2014, no. 4 (2014): CD005451, https://doi.org/10.1002/14651858.CD005451.pub3.

There are other seizure medications that effectively treat nerve pain. Chief among these are carbamazepine (Tegretol) and oxcarbazepine (Trileptal). In some studies, these are more effective than the first drugs we discussed but also come with less tolerable side effects in rare cases.[96] These drugs can affect blood sodium levels (like SSRIs and SNRIs) in the blood. If this change is significant enough or occurs too rapidly, it can result in severe neurologic effects including coma. Some individuals who take these medications are at increased risk of a rare but serious skin reaction called Stevens-Johnson syndrome. This requires prescribers to start these drugs at low doses and increase them gradually. Finally, these drugs may interact with others that are metabolized in the liver, including oral contraceptive pills, blood thinners like warfarin, some antibiotics, and some chemotherapy agents.

Prostaglandins

As if off-label use of medications wasn't already confusing enough, new medications that are modeled after prostaglandins—the same signaling molecules we try to *reduce* with NSAID medications like ibuprofen—may be beneficial in spinal stenosis pain. One subtype in the prostaglandin family, represented by limaprost and misoprostol, may actually improve pain better than some typical nerve pain medications.[97] Because of

---

96 S. Criscuolo et al., "Oxcarbazepine Monotherapy in Postherpetic Neuralgia Unresponsive to Carbamazepine and Gabapentin," *Acta Neurologica Scandinavica* 111, no. 4 (2005): 229–232, https://doi.org/10.1111/j.1600-0404.2005.00300.x; P. Magenta et al., "Oxcarbazepine Is Effective and Safe in the Treatment of Neuropathic Pain: Pooled Analysis of Seven Clinical Studies," *Neurological Sciences* 26, no. 4 (October 2005): 218–226, https://doi.org/10.1007/s10072-005-0464-z.

97 Austin Marcolina et al., "Lumbar Spinal Stenosis and Potential Management with Prostaglandin E1 Analogs," *American Journal of Physical Medicine & Rehabilitation* 100, no. 3 (March 2021): 297–302, https://doi.org/10.1097/PHM.0000000000001620.

how they work, they are not recommended for individuals who are pregnant or plan to become pregnant.

Capsaicin—Feel the Burn!

Serotonin and norepinephrine reduce the pain signal as it's traveling to the brain. The other logical place to interfere with pain signals is the initial detection of the painful stimulus. For example, if you cut your finger, the nerves in your finger are first to detect this injury. They relay the information to the spinal cord and then the brain. Serotonin and norepinephrine send a "quiet down" signal back toward the spot in the spine that received the pain signal. But there are other chemicals that transmit the pain sensation earlier in the process. One of these is called "Substance P." This spicy protein is where capsaicin comes in.

If you aren't familiar with this term, capsaicin is the irritant in chili peppers. It's what makes a pepper spicy, but it also has many health benefits. Applying capsaicin to painful areas essentially uses up all the Substance P in the area. Without this chemical, the nerves are unable to detect the full severity of the painful signal.

The process doesn't occur quickly; it requires many repeated applications to dim the painful signal over time. That means this method isn't effective for acute pain like the finger cut we described above. Instead, capsaicin creams and patches are more effective for painful neuropathy due to conditions like diabetes. The ideal concentration is the strongest you can tolerate.[98]

---

[98] Sheena Derry et al., "Topical Capsaicin (High Concentration) for Chronic Neuropathic Pain in Adults," *Cochrane Database of Systematic Reviews* 1, no. 1 (2017): CD007393, https://doi.org/10.1002/14651858.CD007393.pub4.

The more Substance P you can deplete, the better potential for longer term pain relief.

Pro tip: Wash your hands *thoroughly* after applying, and even then, avoid rubbing your eyes unless you like simulating the feeling of pepper spray in the eyes.

Corticosteroids

Medical professionals often prescribe corticosteroids, or "steroids," like prednisone, methylprednisolone, dexamethasone, triamcinolone, and betamethasone to reduce inflammation and pain. These medicines are effective when taken by mouth or injected directly inside a joint, next to a tendon or ligament, or near compressed or irritated nerves.

The key takeaway is that steroids are useful in the short term but potentially damaging in the long term. When used for short periods of time, these medicines can complement other therapies, allowing you to move more freely and participate in physical therapy. However, for certain conditions, such as chronic low back pain without weakness in the legs (to indicate nerve involvement), research has shown that steroids are often not more effective than a placebo in improving pain. However, if nerve compression *with* inflammation is the source of pain, epidural steroid injections next to the nerve may help rapidly reduce leg pain and short-term disability.[99] Frequent, long-term, or high-dose use in joints may relieve arthritis pain but could speed up cartilage breakdown.

The trade-off is kind of like that scene in *Varsity Blues*. For

---

99 Crystian B. Oliveira et al., "Epidural Corticosteroid Injections for Sciatica: An Abridged Cochrane Systematic Review and Meta-Analysis," *Spine* 45, no. 21 (2020): E1405–E1415, https://doi.org/10.1097/BRS.0000000000003651.

those who missed this classic 1990s coming-of-age movie, Paul Walker's character is a talented quarterback who suffers a knee injury. His coaches, in an attempt to keep him in the game, give him a knee injection of some unknown substance. He is able to go back out to play but ends up paying a greater cost in the long run due to a more permanent knee injury. In reality, this was probably just a numbing medication like lidocaine, and his long-term injury was simply from no longer having pain to remind him to protect his knee. For this comparison, pretend he exchanged short-term pain relief for long-term cartilage damage. In reality, this trade-off would occur over the course of months or years and likely only really happen with repeated injections.

Spinal stenosis is a condition in which the space around the spinal cord is so narrow it compresses the nerve fibers. When this is the cause of pain, steroid injections may be considered for some patients, but response is inconsistent.[100] Special testing may determine if injections are likely to be successful, but this isn't routinely performed ahead of time.[101]

You and your treatment team must always consider the long-term plan when relying on a short-term remedy like steroids for pain and inflammation. These medications are generally safe and effective for short, infrequent courses of treatment. Repeat injections can diminish effectiveness and even potentially worsen the underlying issue. For example, repeat injections

---

100 Roger Chou et al., "Epidural Corticosteroid Injections for Radiculopathy and Spinal Stenosis: A Systematic Review and Meta-Analysis," *Annals of Internal Medicine* 163, no. 5 (2015): 373–381, https://doi.org/10.7326/M15-0934; Massimiliano Carassiti et al., "Epidural Steroid Injections for Low Back Pain: A Narrative Review," *International Journal of Environmental Research and Public Health* 19, no. 1 (2022): 231, https://doi.org/10.3390/ijerph19010231.

101 Chung-Kuang Lin et al., "Predicting Response to Epidural Steroid Injections for Lumbar Spinal Stenosis with Biomarkers and Electromyography," *PM & R* 12, no. 7 (July 2020): 663–670, https://doi.org/10.1002/pmrj.1227.

into joints may speed up the process of osteoarthritis progression. Even steroids by mouth can weaken structures, especially bone density. Recall that Cushing's syndrome can be the result of prolonged steroid use.

Steroids are not a long-term solution and shouldn't be taken lightly. If the goal of treatment is to reduce pain to improve activity levels, steroids effectively target the underlying inflammation. But if the goal is simply to reduce pain until the next injection, you may want to discuss a better, more sustainable long-term plan with your doctor and medical team.

A Trio of Injections

The other injectable treatments we focus on with regards to prehab include platelet-rich plasma (PRP), stem cells, and hyaluronic acid.

PRP, stem cell, and newer related treatments like *exosome therapy* injections are often described as "regenerative medicine" because unlike with corticosteroids that only serve to reduce inflammation, the hope is that these injections will reverse some of the damaged tissue and reduce pain in the process.

Injection preparations vary, but here's a general overview. Platelet-rich plasma is prepared using a blood sample from the patient, which is separated into the different layers of blood (plasma, platelets, white blood cells, and red blood cells.) Depending on the intended mixture, platelets, plasma, and potentially some white blood cells are gathered and put into a syringe.

For stem cell injections, the physician often collects stem cells from a patient's bone marrow or fat cells. These are processed, sometimes mixed with PRP, and then injected at the site of diseased tendons, ligaments, or joints. Research has not concluded which preparation method is most effective and for which problems these treatments work best. These treatments are not currently approved by the Food and Drug Administration (FDA), and thus insurance companies don't typically reimburse them. Costs of each session can range from several hundred dollars into the thousands.

When compared with steroid injections, these treatments may work in situations where steroids aren't effective or suitable. In other situations—plantar fasciitis is a good example—steroids may be more effective than PRP but more limited in their use.[102] PRP and stem cells don't carry the same risks as steroids when repeat injections are involved, meaning they can be used more frequently, provided your budget allows.

Hyaluronic acid is a natural cushion or lubricant found in our joints. When a joint's cartilage has eroded and hyaluronic acid has decreased, it can be helpful to inject this viscous fluid (also called *viscosupplementation*) to increase lubrication and cushioning. Doing so, especially for arthritis, can provide relief of pain and stiffness. Responses vary, and results typically last from a few weeks to a few months. While steroids can speed up the progression of arthritis and orthobiologics may slow it down, hyaluronic acid likely has no effect on the actual arthritis process.

Nonsteroidal Anti-Inflammatory Drugs

It's likely you've taken aspirin or ibuprofen at some point in your life. This class of drugs, known as NSAIDs, reduces pain,

---

[102] Ali Tabrizi et al., "The Effect of Corticosteroid Local Injection Versus Platelet-Rich Plasma for the Treatment of Plantar Fasciitis in Obese Patients: A Single-Blind, Randomized Clinical Trial," *Journal of Foot & Ankle Surgery* 59, no. 1 (January 2020): 64–68, https://doi.org/10.1053/j.jfas.2019.07.004.

fever, and inflammation by blocking specific enzymes in the body (cyclooxygenase or COX) that produce molecules called prostaglandins as part of the body's inflammatory response. By slowing the production of certain prostaglandins, NSAIDs help relieve pain and inflammation.

Prostaglandins aren't all bad and play vital roles in blood vessel function and protection for the stomach lining. Unlike the other major class of over-the-counter pain relievers, acetaminophen (Tylenol), NSAIDs don't usually harm the liver, but because they slow prostaglandin production, they can be harmful to the stomach, intestines, and kidneys. The same enzymes produce other clotting and artery-modulating compounds, which also relates to some unintended side effects.

Some medical professionals are cautious about using NSAIDs for pain relief after surgery (especially orthopedic or spine) because animal studies have suggested they might impair the healing process. Our bodies use inflammation to recruit healing factors, so dampening the signal dampens the healing process. COX enzymes also affect how platelets function, and inhibiting them may increase your risk of bleeding—maybe you've heard that aspirin is a "blood thinner." However, studies in humans have muddied the waters; some show no effect on healing, while others suggest extended NSAID use may mess with bone healing after fractures.

Some doctors may prescribe acetaminophen and short-term opioid pain medication instead of NSAIDs to avoid any potential risk. Other doctors prefer to use NSAIDs that are more "selective" and have a lower risk of causing stomach and kidney problems. With this greater "selectively" for certain COX subtypes, clotting risk can *increase* and contribute to risk of heart attacks and strokes.

NSAIDs aren't risk free, but they are important pain medications. Injectable NSAIDs like ketorolac may be used instead of corticosteroids for similar benefit with lower risk of cartilage damage in joints.[103] Patients on long-term NSAIDs for chronic pain can reduce stomach and intestinal risk by taking acid-blocking medications. These individuals should also drink plenty of fluids to minimize impact on the kidneys. Individuals with blood vessel disease or prior heart attacks or strokes may have lower risk of complications with nonselective NSAIDS like naproxen instead of celecoxib. This is a nuanced conversation to have with your prehab team.

Opioid Pain Medication

In the 1990s and 2000s, physicians prescribed opioid pain medications to patients with acute and chronic pain much more freely than they do today…maybe you see where this is going. That "casual" practice led to the opioid epidemic, with effects we're still witnessing, despite current stricter guidelines.

Now, patients with severe, acute pain are having trouble managing their pain, especially if they've received opioids in the past, built a tolerance to these medications, and now require higher doses for the same relief. Current rules have likely helped prevent new addiction and misuse, but hesitancy has also made some medical professionals uncertain about when opioid medications are appropriate and the reasonable doses.

Opioids are most commonly prescribed for cancer-associated pain, given its character and severity. Patients may reasonably

---

103 Jaime L. Bellamy et al., "Economic Impact of Ketorolac vs Corticosteroid Intra-Articular Knee Injections for Osteoarthritis: A Randomized, Double-Blind, Prospective Study," *Journal of Arthroplasty* 31, no. 9 Supplement (September 2016): 293–297, https://doi.org/10.1016/j.arth.2016.05.015; Kevin Jurgensmeier et al., "Intra-Articular Injections of the Hip and Knee with Triamcinolone vs Ketorolac: A Randomized Controlled Trial," *Journal of Arthroplasty* 36, no. 2 (February 2021): 416–422, https://doi.org/10.1016/j.arth.2020.08.036.

expect opioid medications when undergoing cancer prehabilitation and after orthopedic and spine surgeries, amputation, and organ transplants. Other procedures like bariatric surgery and cesarean section may also warrant opioids.

In a pain treatment program with multiple medication types, certain opioids are appropriate for moderate or severe pain when other medications aren't controlling pain. When warranted, there's a time and a place for opioids, and individuals shouldn't feel guilty for taking them. Postoperative pain can be debilitating, and opioids may be critical medications to make physical or occupational therapy even possible during recovery. The benefits of therapy participation greatly outweigh the risk of short, low-dose courses of opioids for most patients, but respect for their risks may lower risk of dependence.

Naltrexone

In low doses, naltrexone is primarily used to reverse the actions of opioid medications or to prevent their activity in patients trying to stay sober. The natural opioid system in the body doesn't function in a black-or-white, all-or-nothing manner. For example, at low doses, opioids control acute sources of pain. At high doses over longer periods, opioids like oxycodone, morphine, hydrocodone, and heroin actually *increase* pain perception, which contributes to the dependence on these medications.

High doses of naltrexone blindly block the different opioid receptors and even reduce the pleasurable effects of alcohol and food. As introduced earlier, when paired with bupropion, this is one way naltrexone helps patients lose weight. However, low doses of naltrexone may regulate inflammation in the brain and spinal cord by binding and blocking receptors on microglia cells.[104] At the same time, the blockade of opioid receptors actually causes the body to increase activity in the natural "endogenous" opioid system. Instead of taking opioids, low doses of naltrexone trigger the body to produce its own.

Think of this like a manager who transfers staff to an overwhelmed department. The low-dose naltrexone is like you rounding up the other workers and shoving them in a closet so that when the manager arrives, the department looks critically understaffed. To correct this, suddenly he calls in people from their day off to pitch in and, voila, now you've got more hands on deck. This is how blocking the opioid receptor leads to increased natural pain relief.

Researchers are studying low-dose naltrexone to treat conditions with inflammatory components—inflammatory bowel disease, multiple sclerosis, complex regional pain syndrome (CRPS, formerly known as reflex sympathetic dystrophy, or RSD), and fibromyalgia.[105] The current evidence is mixed but promising. Low-dose naltrexone typically has minor side effects, so it can be a great add-on to pain treatment regimens for patients in prehabilitation programs, as long as they aren't taking opioids.

---

104 Phillip S. Kim and Michael A. Fishman, "Low-Dose Naltrexone for Chronic Pain: Update and Systemic Review," *Current Pain and Headache Reports* 24, no. 10 (2020): 64, https://doi.org/10.1007/s11916-020-00898-0.

105 Claire E. Parker et al., "Low Dose Naltrexone for Induction of Remission in Crohn's Disease," *Cochrane Database of Systematic Reviews* 4, no. 4 (2018): CD010410, https://doi.org/10.1002/14651858.CD010410.pub3; Amol Soin et al., "Low-Dose Naltrexone Use for Patients with Chronic Regional Pain Syndrome: A Systematic Literature Review," *Pain Physician* 24, no. 4 (July 2021): E393–E406, https://pubmed.ncbi.nlm.nih.gov/34213865/; Luke Parkitny and Jarred Younger, "Reduced Pro-Inflammatory Cytokines After Eight Weeks of Low-Dose Naltrexone for Fibromyalgia," *Biomedicines* 5, no. 2 (2017): 16, https://doi.org/10.3390/biomedicines5020016; Ariadna Colomer-Carbonell et al., "Study Protocol for a Randomised, Double-Blinded, Placebo-Controlled Phase III Trial Examining the Add-On Efficacy, Cost-Utility and Neurobiological Effects of Low-Dose Naltrexone (LDN) in Patients with Fibromyalgia (INNOVA Study)," *BMJ Open* 12, no. 1 (2022): 1–11, e055351, https://doi.org/10.1136/bmjopen-2021-055351.

Cannabis

Cannabis, also known as marijuana, is a plant with thousands of years of global cultural use that contains several compounds with biological effects. The two primary compounds are tetrahydrocannabinol (THC) and cannabidiol (CBD), though dozens of cannabinoids exist in the cannabis plant.

THC has psychoactive properties that make users feel "high," while CBD produces subtler effects. Because of these and other chemical compounds, cannabis may have several potential roles for individuals with different issues like pain, nausea, and insomnia. Cannabis overall has apparent sleep-promoting activity, but THC may impair sleep quality while CBD likely does not.[106] Studies have shown that cannabis may be beneficial alone or with other medications for managing chronic pain. For acute pain, such as after surgery, cannabis can increase the relief provided by opioids.[107] In such cases, this allows a lower opioid dose to control pain with fewer side effects.

During prehab or preop, recreational or medical cannabis may have some risk, and some surgical programs require abstinence for *at least* seventy-two hours before general anesthesia. It can affect blood flow, body temperature regulation, and drug metabolism.[108]

---

[106] Kimberly A. Babson et al., "Cannabis, Cannabinoids, and Sleep: a Review of the Literature," *Current Psychiatry Reports* 19, no. 4 (April 2017): 23, https://doi.org/10.1007/s11920-017-0775-9.

[107] Pierre Beaulieu, "Cannabinoids and Acute/Postoperative Pain Management," *Pain* 162, no. 8 (August 2021): 2309, https://doi.org/10.1097/j.pain.0000000000002294.

[108] Marco Echeverria-Villalobos et al., "Perioperative Care of Cannabis Users: A Comprehensive Review of Pharmacological and Anesthetic Considerations," *Journal of Clinical Anesthesia* 57 (November 2019): 41–49, https://doi.org/10.1016/j.jclinane.2019.03.011.

Psychedelic Medicine

Pain and depression are two major things to monitor in this pillar, but so are adjustment disorders like anxiety and post-traumatic stress disorder (PTSD). These are especially relevant during cancer prehab or after receiving a terminal diagnosis, and psychedelic medicines are proving to be highly therapeutic in this area. Major universities and hospital systems around the world are studying psychedelic substances like psilocybin, LSD, ketamine, and others as potential treatments.

Decades ago, psilocybin and LSD were expected to be the next big things in psychiatry, but because of cultural elements, they were classified as Schedule I substances, incorrectly deemed to have no medical benefit and high risk for harm. Ketamine avoided this defamation because of its use as a surgical anesthetic. Because of this acceptance, it's the first psychedelic approved for treating depression (as a slightly different formulation) and is also prescribed off-label for chronic pain.

Ketamine and psilocybin are unique relative to SSRIs and SNRIs in how they treat depression because their effects are nearly immediate. Traditional depression medications may take weeks or months to achieve similar benefits. These treatments may even improve depression or chronic pain that resists other treatments. For example, researchers found that ketamine significantly reduced nerve and non-nerve chronic pain including all types of CRPs, conditions that are notoriously difficult to treat.[109] Ketamine and psilocybin may each play a role in break-

---

[109] Dermot P. Maher et al., "Intravenous Ketamine Infusions for Neuropathic Pain Management: A Promising Therapy in Need of Optimization," *Anesthesia & Analgesia* 124, no. 2 (February 2017): 661–674, https://doi.org/10.1213/ANE.0000000000001787; Vwaire Orhurhu et al., "Ketamine Infusions for Chronic Pain: A Systematic Review and Meta-analysis of Randomized Controlled Trials," *Anesthesia & Analgesia* 129, no. 1 (July 2019): 241–254, https://doi.org/10.1213/ANE.0000000000004185.

through treatments for "treatment resistant depression," or depression that doesn't respond well to common treatments.

Psilocybin is the psychoactive ingredient in psychedelic mushrooms. It has promoted large reductions in anxiety and depression often, with rare serious side effects.[110] In a study comparing psilocybin to the SSRI escitalopram, psilocybin was found to be just as effective in reducing depression severity after six weeks, but with a much quicker response and fewer side effects overall.[111] However, some studies show that like with traditional antidepressants, risk of suicide increases early in treatment in rare cases.

The ultimate goal is to gain more knowledge on how different psychedelics can be used in medicine. Most psychedelics act through nearly identical pathways, but they can have slightly varying use cases—some may work better with therapy while others might be relatively better at treating addiction.[112] Research has its limitations because patients can usually tell if they've been given the active drug or a placebo. This makes it difficult to determine exactly how effective a psychedelic is for a specific purpose. That being said, these drugs can be highly effective for treating depression, pain, and anxiety, even when other medications have little impact.

---

[110] Simon B. Goldberg et al., "The Experimental Effects of Psilocybin on Symptoms of Anxiety and Depression: A Meta-Analysis," *Psychiatry Research* 284 (February 2020): 112749, https://doi.org/10.1016/j.psychres.2020.112749.

[111] Robin Carhart-Harris et al., "Trial of Psilocybin Versus Escitalopram for Depression," *New England Journal of Medicine* 384, no. 15 (2021): 1402–1411, https://doi.org/10.1056/nejmoa2032994.

[112] Yuan Yao et al., "Efficacy and Safety on Psychedelics for the Treatment of Mental Disorders: A Systematic Review and Meta-Analysis," *Psychiatry Research* 335 (May 2024): 115886, https://doi.org/10.1016/j.psychres.2024.115886.

MAYBE THERE'S A BETTER WAY!

When it comes to medication treatment plans, a worthy goal is elegantly limiting the number of medications a patient needs. This can be done by removing medications with negligible benefit, or drugs that are needed to reduce unintended side effects of others. For example, some patients may take medications that worsen control of diabetes simply because they had already been on them for years prior to being diagnosed with diabetes. Now, partially because of these medications, they need other drugs to keep their blood sugar under control. Changing the first drug could lead to needing less of the others.

Our goal, in prehab and in general, isn't exactly to prescribe however many drugs are needed to completely eliminate symptoms or disease. It's to prescribe the fewest possible that offer the best results with the least side effects. This section will focus on potential switches from medications that may contribute to unintended side effects. As with *every* section of this book, don't make any of the described changes without the recommendation and guidance of your personal medical team. Just because a medication is in this section doesn't imply it was an oversight or mistake—this drug might work the best out of all options for an intended purpose. The following is for educational purposes.

Antipsychotics

Some pathways that mediate the effects of antipsychotics are also involved in appetite and energy regulation. That means these drugs often come with metabolic side effects. Newer-generation antipsychotics were developed with a goal of avoiding some of the movement-related side effects in the original drugs. Like so much in the medicine world, that meant a trade-off. Patients on drugs like risperidone, clozapine, olanzapine, and quetiapine often had to accept weight gain and risk of diabetes to control psychotic symptoms.

There's some good news. Newer drugs like paliperidone, lurasidone, aripiprazole, cariprazine, and others have a lower risk of these metabolic side effects. In many cases, medical teams and patients prefer not to rock the boat by switching off a regimen that works. If this isn't the case, or in cases of intolerable metabolic symptoms, transitioning to a newer drug may provide a different path forward that's more sustainable.

Antidepressants

A couple of antidepressants, such as bupropion and potentially fluoxetine, contribute to weight loss, but most antidepressants come with a risk of weight gain. The exact reason isn't clear because these drugs typically work with multiple neurotransmitters. Plus, appetite's effect on mood is a heavy contributor to weight gain or loss. For example, a person with depression might have a diminished or high appetite. Treating depression usually makes appetite trend back toward the average—someone with a low appetite might increase food intake or vice versa. These medications usually stimulate appetite less than antipsychotics, but individual experiences can vary.

Some antidepressants are more associated with weight gain than others. Tricyclic antidepressants like amitriptyline and nortriptyline, MAO inhibitors such as phenelzine and atypical antidepressants like mirtazapine are more likely to cause weight gain than newer drug classes like SSRIs and SNRIs. However, paroxetine (SSRI) and venlafaxine (SNRI) may also cause weight gain more than their counterparts in the same classes. The key is knowing how these medications will potentially impact appetite and weight and how that could impact a broader prehabilitation regimen.

Diabetes Medications

For the most part (metformin being a notable exception), the original diabetes medications worked by increasing the body's production of insulin or making it more effective. Insulin is the hormone that tells certain cells to take glucose (sugar) out of the blood, but it also tells those cells *not* to burn fat.

As a result, these early medications promoted weight gain and, over time, made it more difficult to control diabetes without any other changes as insulin requirements increased. However, metformin is one of the oldest non-insulin medications that even has the ability to promote weight loss for some patients. As for the biggest weight-gain culprits, insulin, sulfonylureas like glipizide, and meglitinides like repaglinide are at the top of the list. Medications like the GLP-1 receptor agonists (liraglutide, semaglutide, and related medications like tirzepatide) promote the most weight loss while also controlling short-term blood sugar. In the long term, weight loss also indirectly aids blood sugar control.

> This does not mean that low-carb (read: low insulin) diets are the only effective diets for weight loss in individuals without diabetes. Nutrition science and medicine is never this straightforward.

Hormones and Anti-Hormonal Medications

Cortisol is a naturally occurring steroid hormone in the body that directly leads to high blood sugar and fat gain while contributing to muscle wasting over time. Corticosteroid medications that work similarly to cortisol come with the same risk. This is worth being aware of, especially during prehab. In cases with certain autoimmune conditions, after organ transplant, or in situations where the goal is to quickly reduce immune system activity, steroids are typically go-to medications because they act rapidly and predictably.

When it comes to sex hormones (estrogen, progesterone, and testosterone), medications that either affect hormone levels or mimic hormone effects can impact weight and metabolic health. Progesterone-related drugs may cause weight gain and fluid retention. However, medications used to reduce estrogen and testosterone activity—used for cases like treating breast or prostate cancer—may also promote an unhealthy metabolic picture. That's because estrogen and testosterone are critical for muscle building, bone density, and energy levels. Blocking these hormones can make the opposite effect occur.[113] Keeping cancer in check understandably outweighs these risks, traditionally.

Blood Pressure Medications

It's a safe bet that if medications work in the opposite direction of weight-loss medications, they'll likely promote weight gain. Certain medications work within the sympathetic (fight-or-

---

[113] N. Pemmaraju et al., "Retrospective Review of Male Breast Cancer Patients: Analysis of Tamoxifen-Related Side-Effects," *Annals of Oncology* 23, no. 6 (June 2012): 1471–1474, https://doi.org/10.1093/annonc/mdr459; Kristian Buch et al., "Effect of Chemotherapy and Aromatase Inhibitors in the Adjuvant Treatment of Breast Cancer on Glucose and Insulin Metabolism—A Systematic Review," *Cancer Medicine* 8, no. 1 (January 2019): 238–245, https://doi.org/10.1002/cam4.1911.

flight) pathways, but beta blockers that do not selectively target *only* heart tissue (metoprolol) are likely to have negative side effects.

Propranolol works in this manner by blocking multiple receptors in this pathway throughout the body, associating its chronic use with weight gain and diabetes.[114] To make this worse, the purpose of these medications is to lower blood pressure by decreasing how hard the heart is beating, which means they reduce a person's exercise intensity. Other blood pressure classes like calcium channel blockers come with less risk of weight gain, and if weight gain occurs, it could be partially due to water retention in the legs instead of predominantly body fat.

Antiseizure Drugs and Mood Stabilizers

Original antiseizure medications (valproic acid or divalproex, among others) have well-known weight gain effects when used for long periods. Gabapentinoids like gabapentin and pregabalin still have a (lower) risk of weight gain, even when used for nerve pain.

Lithium is a naturally occurring mineral and has been a mood-stabilizing medication for centuries, but it may also cause weight gain when used at a dosage required to manage bipolar disorder.[115] On the other hand, seizure medications like phenytoin (Dilantin), levetiracetam (Keppra), and lamotrigine (Lamictal) are more weight neutral. Zonisamide and topiramate may promote weight loss.

---

[114] T. Pischon and A. M. Sharma, "Use of Beta-Blockers in Obesity Hypertension: Potential Role of Weight Gain," *Obesity Reviews* 2, no. 4 (November 2001): 275–280, https://doi.org/10.1046/j.1467-789X.2001.00044.x.

[115] T. Baptista et al., "Lithium and Body Weight Gain," *Pharmacopsychiatry* 28, no. 2 (1995): 35–44, https://doi.org/10.1055/s-2007-979586.

Knowing each of these medications by heart and being able to recite how they work and their potential side effects isn't the point of this chapter. Neither is having an exhaustive understanding of every screening and test a physician might use when you walk into the doctor's office. But if you're reading this in preparation for prehabilitation due to a major procedure or treatment, odds are some of the information applies to your situation.

Knowing what you're getting into and where the journey leads can be the difference between a life worsened by anxiety and a feeling of relative calm and control. You don't need to second-guess your medical team at every turn, but it's also nice to understand what they're doing and why. The questions doctors ask us and tests they perform have a massive impact on the medications and supplements prescribed later, and this is so easy to overlook. Understanding how everything is related can make a person more confident in managing their unique medication blend, and more confident in their prehabilitation program.

ACTION POINTS

- "Diagnostics" are for gaining an understanding of a patient's unique history, physical examination, blood testing, and lab work. These provide physicians with the complete picture, which becomes vital when prescribing treatments and medications.
- Medications are rapidly advancing, with many exciting breakthroughs on the horizon. That being said, a pill or injection alone will rarely—or never—fix all of a person's ailments. While medications continue to improve, they still come with side effects and may require behavioral changes of the patient.

- Some methods that offer benefit or relief from a condition don't require pharmaceutically synthesized drugs. Tools like capsaicin, cannabis, and psychedelic medicine have shown real benefit in treating pain, anxiety, and depression and are being standardized into medical treatments.
- Old medications with less benefit or unintended side effects can, when possible, be replaced by more efficient strategies that can potentially even help multiple diseases at once. This is particularly true with antipsychotics, antidepressants, diabetes medications, hormones, blood pressure medications, and antiseizure drugs.

PART II

CHAPTER 3

ORTHOPEDIC PREHABILITATION

ODDS ARE, YOU OR SOMEONE YOU KNOW WILL HAVE A JOINT replaced or any type of back surgery at some point in your life. Many of us become tolerant of daily pain, but there comes a point when the pain progresses or its simple presence takes too high of a toll on our lifestyle. That's when treatment enters the picture.

This chapter's focus is on prehab for joint replacements and back surgery for when you've reached this stage. Surgery is a major undertaking, which is precisely why we take preparation so seriously. Traditionally, a person suffering from orthopedic pain starts with oral medications. When those alone aren't enough or you've got a proactive approach, physical therapy enters the picture to complement treatment outcomes. Should these remain inadequate, this can lead to targeted injections, often followed by more or different physical therapy. Typically, all those measures would fail before surgery would become a major consideration. In cases that involve nagging pain, we want to do everything we can to avoid surgery or delay time before requiring it as much as possible.

Like nearly everything in medicine, a person's treatment in this situation isn't one size fits all. Depending on age and severity, there is most definitely a point when an individual starts becoming a "worse candidate" for surgery. While orthopedic surgeries may occur before conservative options are completely exhausted, I've had at least as many cases of a patient wishing they'd gotten the joint replaced years earlier. A fine balance exists here. For instance, if a person in their late sixties is *clearly* going to need a hip replacement at some point, it might make more sense to have that done while they're relatively young. These surgeries often have fewer complications, and frankly, the patient has more time to utilize the fresh new anatomy.

Whatever the decision and regardless of the type of orthopedic surgery, prehabilitation can play a huge role in preparation, promote faster recovery, and improve quality of life prior to surgery.

TREATMENT TEAM AND HELPFUL TERMINOLOGY

Preparing for surgery can be an overwhelming series of consultations, clearances, and tests. When it comes to everything related to joint replacement and spinal surgery, this chapter will illustrate what you need to know and how best to prepare.

Joints "electively" need replacing when arthritis becomes too severe and painful to bear. As this pain leads to inactivity, individuals become prone to weight gain and greater difficulty controlling diseases like diabetes, which promotes further weight gain in a vicious cycle. Conditions like spinal stenosis (the spinal central canal becoming too narrow and "pinching" the spinal cord or nerves) and radiculopathy (when the space around the nerve exiting the spine is too narrow) also contribute to pain and inactivity.

The bottom line: it's hard to stay healthy and keep weight under control if you're in too much pain to move.

SURGERY TEAM

After an initial visit with a primary care provider (PCP), you may have several new faces to learn. The first could very well be an orthopedic surgeon or neurosurgeon (for spine surgery). This doctor may also go by "orthopedist." Note: spine surgeons can be specialist orthopedic surgeons or neurosurgeons, and neither is necessarily "better."

PAIN MANAGEMENT

A pain management specialist usually enters the picture around the same time. These professionals are trained to perform more advanced procedures than your typical orthopedist or PCP, including nerve blocks to different joints, injections into the space around the nerves leaving the spine under fluoroscopic (special X-ray) guidance, and ultrasound-guided procedures for surrounding tendon or ligament disease.

Managing pain is a huge part of prehab because although staying active is incredibly important, patients often think pain signifies they are causing further damage. Controlling pain and staying active will likely lead to less pain overall, and after surgery, these patients tend to have much better outcomes. That being said, pain management providers can be nonsurgical specialists such as a physical medicine & rehabilitation (PM&R) specialist (physiatrist) or anesthesiologist.

PHYSICAL AND OCCUPATIONAL THERAPISTS

Physical therapists design treatments to improve strength, flexibility, mobility, and endurance. This might involve therapies to improve range of motion, balance, and coordination, as well as ways to manage pain and swelling. Physical therapy can also help patients address the side effects of joint and spinal disease including weakness and pain in surrounding joints, bones, and nerves. The therapy team anticipates side effects of medical/surgical treatments for arthritis and spinal disorders and designs prehab programs that will directly reduce their negative impact and compensate for negative effects that might develop.

On the other hand, occupational therapy focuses on helping patients regain independence in their daily activities through new modified ways to perform tasks like dressing, grooming, and cooking. Occupational therapy can also help patients deal with the challenges of returning to work or other activities after treatment.

CARE OVERVIEW

The average patient doesn't immediately leap to a consultation with a surgeon the instant they have joint pain. A PCP's opinion is usually the first a person receives—diagnostic workup and treatment methods that resolve pain and defer surgery are a priority. They will often prescribe a nonsteroidal anti-inflammatory drug (NSAID), or in some cases a short course of steroids like prednisone or methylprednisolone (Medrol). For arthritis or back pain conditions, gone are the days of liberal opioid prescriptions, and for good reason. Opioids don't fix the problem, and they even make a person *more* pain-sensitive after frequent use. NSAIDs and steroids may also be prescribed after an evaluation of chronic neck or back pain, especially when there's high suspicion of a pinched nerve or spinal stenosis.

Treating pain in this way is done to delay or avoid surgery by making the pain bearable enough to resume physical activity, and physical therapy is often part of this process. Here's something you should know about pain management: *completely curing pain isn't the goal in most cases because it's often unrealistic.* Instead, prescribers provide pain relief to allow exercise participation and physical therapy to strengthen supporting muscles and restore "normal" joint movements to balance the load off joints and the spine. Exercise directly and indirectly also lowers inflammation, which may relieve pain and helps fight metabolic diseases like diabetes. The physical therapy route can slow worsening of the underlying issue while reducing symptoms.

For some, pain and disability persist despite best efforts to reduce them. If initial conservative measures fail, a patient may be referred to an orthopedic surgeon or physiatrist. Physiatrists (not podiatrist, psychiatrist, or physical therapist...I've been called all these and more) specialize in nonsurgical care of neurologic (brain, spinal cord, and nerves) and musculoskeletal (muscles, bones, joints, and connective tissue) systems with training in joint and spine injections and methods for advanced pain control. Pain medicine specialists are typically physiatrists or anesthesiologists who undergo an additional year of fellowship training focusing exclusively on diagnosing and treating (i.e., advanced injections and outpatient procedures) pain conditions.

A physiatrist might add to medications prescribed by a PCP with things like serotonin and norepinephrine reuptake inhibitors (SNRIs), especially when the pain has a mood or nerve component. For individuals with joint disease who haven't recently had a steroid, PRP, or hyaluronic acid injection in the joint, the physiatrist might recommend one of these for pain relief. Steroid injections can also be appropriate for back pain with symptoms of nerve involvement. An injection next to the nerves in and around the spine can reduce acute or active inflammation and pain.

These measures may buy months or years of relief, but they usually can't don't reverse the damage or stop new damage from being caused. This scenario would lead to an eventual consultation with surgeons.

SURGERY CONSULTATION

Prehabilitation begins when a person has reached the point where surgery is a real possibility. For individuals without other significant medical issues, the preoperative period may be short and sweet. It could be as simple as a generic plan that reminds a person to "Eat well and exercise!"

This plan quickly becomes more structured when things like a high body mass index (BMI), hard-to-control diabetes, sleep apnea, lung disease, or other complicating factors are in play. Sleep apnea and lung disease, for instance, can make anesthesia risky, and this is when a surgeon may be reluctant to operate without some preparation.

These concerns aren't meant to discriminate. Something like BMI, which is a simple and crude snapshot of a person's health, likely won't be enough by itself to determine whether or not a person is fit for surgery. Surgeons often have an upper limit on a patient's BMI (often thirty-five to forty) before they become unwilling to perform a surgery because a high BMI *does* often point to other risks lurking below the surface. These risk factors increase the odds of complications and make a good outcome—in our case, a well-healing new joint—less likely.

If you've struggled with "weight"—formally, the legitimate chronic disease of obesity—then preoperative health improvements will prioritize a few core areas of our prehab pillars from Chapter 1. What follows is how the prehabilitation pillars can be specifically tailored to orthopedic surgery beyond "just lose weight."

PREHABILITATION PILLARS: JOINT REPLACEMENT AND SPINE

As we've discussed, although a handful of basic concepts overlap between diagnoses in this book, the preparation for one type of procedure may be quite different from the next.

EXERCISE

With joint and spine surgeries, one factor that makes them unique is how patients compensate for the injured area. Imagine a person with really bad knee pain in their right knee that has lasted for months or years. You would expect this person to favor their left side, putting all their weight on those muscles and joints.

Years of limping, leaning, or neglecting a limb can cause an imbalance that should likely be corrected, especially if it has become its own "pain generator." This imbalance means that the body is no longer functionally symmetrical, and asymmetry can cause new pain in the overburdened joints and connective tissues. It's common for back pain to get worse or for a good knee to start hurting because it's doing more work than it should.

A major part of the exercise portion of prehab and therapy involves unlearning bad habits and, ideally, strengthening the muscles around a bad joint. For those awaiting spine surgery (particularly in the low back), this often means more leg exercises, since they may have compensated by limiting all activity.

For both joint and spine prehab patients, low weight or low impact exercises like aquatic therapy or "zero-G"/anti-gravity ("unweighting") treadmills can improve aerobic conditioning without making pain worse.

Muscle strengthening is crucial but requires care and proper planning. For individuals without joint or back pain, compound exercises like squats are a great way to increase metabolism and build muscle. Because they work several muscles unlike single-joint ("open chain") exercises, they are more time efficient and better at building muscle throughout functional groups—i.e., strengthening the quads, hamstrings, and calf muscles simultaneously. However, these exercises are limited by the weakest link in the chain. If a bad knee can only bear twenty pounds of weight, compound movements like squats are nearly out of the question.

That's where something like blood-flow restriction (BFR) training can be very helpful. Like we discussed in Chapter 1, BFR restricts blood circulation out of the limb doing exercise. This is kind of like that limb firing off a flare gun to attract the cavalry for maximum healing power. When done properly, BFR allows you to "trick" the muscle into thinking it worked harder than it did.

Isometric exercise is another way to get stronger and build muscle while moving a painful joint or spine as little as possible. This involves getting into a position where the muscle is working to keep you in that position—a plank or wall sit, holding a pushup position, etc. Because the joints aren't moving, you can get some of the benefit from the exercise with less pain.

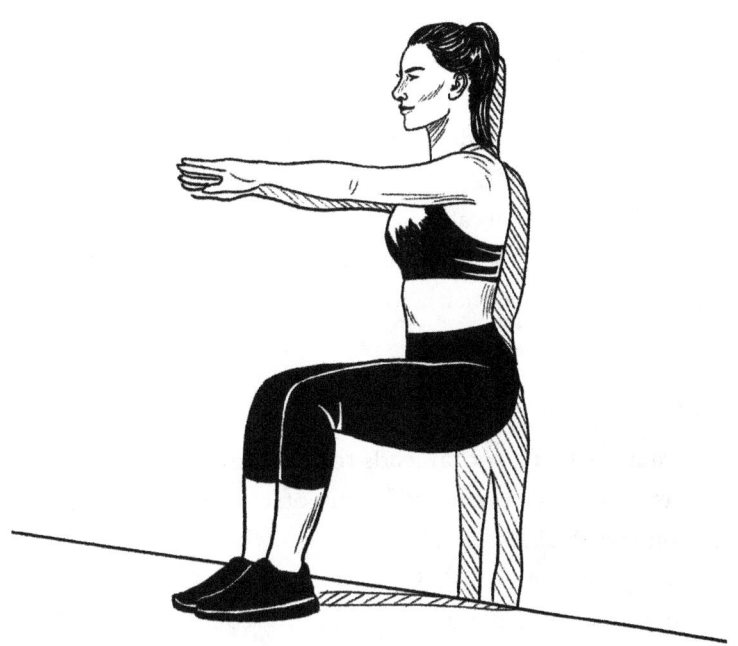

Demonstration of isometric exercise such as a wall sit

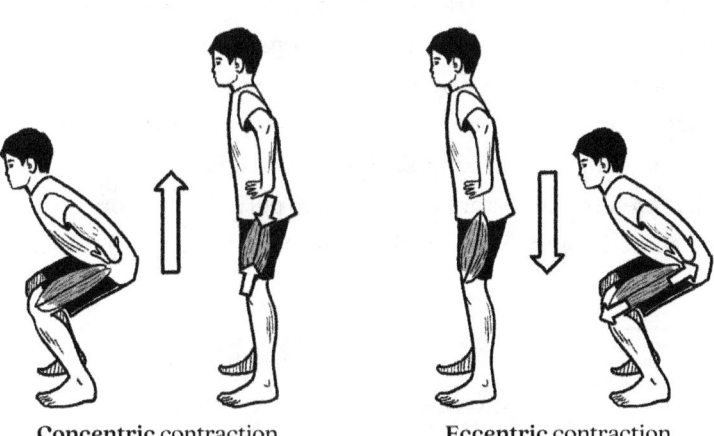

Concentric contraction **Eccentric** contraction

Demonstration of concentric versus eccentric portion of repetitions

Also keep in mind that patients with hip or knee arthritis or spinal stenosis are at a higher risk of falls.[116] Coupling resistance training with balance training before joint replacement decreases the risk of falls and also improves resilience to trauma if they should fall.[117] As able, a foundation of low-impact walking throughout the whole program can function as complementary aerobic and pain desensitization therapy as well.

LIFESTYLE

One main risk factor that leads to many of the complications on the surgery side tends to be out-of-control blood sugar. A person with diabetes, in combination with exercise, may benefit from either a low-carb diet or a supervised fasting program. The objective, regardless of diet type, is to control the metabolic side of things within a (typically) limited timeline. This can be a drastic dietary overhaul, which is often necessary since we're talking weeks or a few months to prepare, not years. Both low-carb and fasting programs, as mentioned earlier, can speed up the effects of exercise and medications in quickly controlling blood sugar. Elevated sugar in the blood increases the risk of surgical infections because sugar is bacteria food.

Smoking and drinking alcohol are two other lifestyle changes that are very important in the prehab period before orthopedic or spine surgery. Smoking is undeniably bad for your overall

---

116 Adam L. Doré et al., "Lower-Extremity Osteoarthritis and the Risk of Falls in a Community-Based Longitudinal Study of Adults with and without Osteoarthritis," *Arthritis Care & Research* 67, no. 5 (May 2015): 593–738, https://doi.org/10.1002/acr.22499; Ho-Joong Kim et al., "The Risk Assessment of a Fall in Patients with Lumbar Spinal Stenosis," *Spine* 36, no. 9 (2011): E588–E592, https://doi.org/10.1097/BRS.0b013e3181f92d8e.

117 Jennifer E. Layne and Miriam E. Nelson, "The Effects of Progressive Resistance Training on Bone Density: A Review," *Medicine & Science in Sports & Exercise* 31, no. 1 (January 1999): 25–30, https://doi.org/10.1097/00005768-199901000-00006.

health, and alcohol is directly bad for exercise recovery, as is being full of "empty" calories.

The recommendations are even connected to the risk factors for developing joint disease, back disease, and arthritis. Our modern lifestyles tend to promote inflammation, and the three things listed above are major contributors. People with joint or back issues are going to be more likely to have a higher BMI and metabolic disease because those two accelerate joint damage and worsen arthritis. Adding smoking or alcohol on top of that just makes the problem worse by turning up the inflammatory heat.

Consider the difference between "fat mass" and "sick fat" diseases. With fat mass diseases, a person carrying more weight is going to put more stress on their joints. Sick fat is the metabolic and inflammatory side of extra weight. Due to this high blood sugar and inflammation, the latter group's joints tend to worsen quicker than someone with "just" the extra impact effect. Think of both diseases as the flint and tinder that create the fire we know as arthritis.

NEUROPSYCHIATRIC

Arguably, our biggest focus within the neuropsych pillar is pain management. In many cases, when dealing with any joint, back, or neck issue, the pain can make sleep or even lying down pretty difficult, leading to poor, fragmented sleep. Sometimes a special bed is needed, but at this stage, it's unlikely to be covered by insurance.

With this in mind, pain control and ensuring patients get quality, consistent sleep go hand in hand. Bad sleep also tends to go along with obesity due to risks of sleep apnea and acid reflux. Add joint or back pain, and it can get even worse.

A more detailed guide to reducing pain and managing sleep can be found in the neuropsychiatric pillar of our prehabilitation overview in Chapter 1. Chapter 2 provides a detailed breakdown of useful medications and potential supplements.

EXPECTATION MANAGEMENT

In some cases, you don't know what you don't know. When it comes to joint and spine surgery, there are a few important points you may not have considered.

We've already touched on this, but it's worth repeating: during prehab and after surgery, the goal of pain control isn't zero pain. It's achieving a tolerable level of pain. Some fortunate patients might experience complete relief from the right mix of pain control methods, but that isn't guaranteed. However, it's reasonable to expect that after dealing with severe pain, you'll be able to endure a much lower level of pain. This "tolerable pain target" is the case when walking a day or so after surgery. Being active as soon as possible helps speed recovery, minimizes complications, and gets you home sooner. So be prepared to have a physical or occupational therapist encouraging you out of bed within twenty-four hours of surgery, provided your blood pressure and oxygen levels are appropriate and stable.

The remaining important points to note all have to deal with ways to put off surgery while making life and pain levels more manageable.

DELAY SURGERY REQUIREMENT

End-stage joint disease is a term for when joints are "bone on bone" *and* have severe pain. Bone on bone isn't a great way to describe arthritis because the real issues are everything that (often, not always) comes along with that. However, I must emphasize, your X-ray (or MRI) is *not* your pain. A "terrible" looking image doesn't mean you must be in worse pain than you are, just as a "moderate" amount of disease doesn't mean you aren't allowed to be in pain. In spine disease, this usually results in severe leg and/or back pain or weakness in those areas. Once you're on the path to end-stage joint disease, few things—if any—will completely change where that path ends. At the time of this writing, while treatments may improve joint or spine health, we don't have a true "fix" to offer, short of surgery when that time comes.

However, that doesn't mean you have to schedule a surgery consultation the moment you read this. Life is busy and complicated. The next question becomes: how do we buy you some time?

Returning to earlier concepts, there are several treatments that can either extend the remaining life of a joint or quiet the pain. In most cases, first line treatments include physical therapy and oral medications like NSAIDs. For some, other medications like SNRIs or gabapentin-related medications are recommended, especially if there is nerve pain like in spinal stenosis or a pinched nerve in the lower back. These drugs manage symptoms, but they won't affect or improve the disease. Some experience profound relief with these, while others do not.

Along those lines, physical therapy usually doesn't change or stop the underlying issue. But depending on how functional you are, it could have the most benefit if it allows you to go from being completely sedentary to a reasonable level of activity. Weight loss also commonly provides relief for joint and lower back pain. Generally, losing 5 to 10 percent of body weight is all that's needed for the start of this benefit. This works fastest and makes the most difference when done through a multimodal diet and exercise plan. Exercise helps lower inflammation, improves chronic disease, and improves body mechanics for "better" movement patterns. Weight loss on its own can also lower inflammation and improve pain sensitivity, especially if diseases like sleep apnea and diabetes also improve.

Often, the next step when trying to delay surgery for shoulder, hip, or knee joints is to undergo joint injections. As detailed earlier, potential injections range between steroids, NSAIDs (ketorolac), and "orthobiologics" (hyaluronic acid, PRP, or stem cells). Steroids cannot be injected long term because they damage cartilage—consider them something that may speed up disease. NSAID injections in a joint may be as effective as steroids with less or minimal impact on cartilage health; this is an ongoing area of research.

Some healthcare providers sell PRP and stem cells as a way to restore joints. For the sake of reasonable expectations, consider them as an option that won't *worsen* the joint while providing pain relief that could potentially last longer than other options. You also have the option to keep using them until they lose their pain-relieving effects. And the pain relief of hyaluronic acid—usually for knees—is likely similar to NSAIDs, although it works in a completely different way. Hyaluronic acid is only FDA approved in knees at the time of this writing. An injection in any other joint will likely be paid for out of pocket.

The next level of invasiveness is nerve blocks and nerve ablations—damaging the nerve on purpose so it can't transmit pain. If a large or small joint has painful arthritis, stopping the function of nerves at that joint will prevent the patient from feeling the arthritis. This is not the same as the process for treating a pinched nerve (described later). Typically, the first step is a chemical block. A pain specialist will inject a numbing medication like lidocaine around the nerve to ensure pain is relieved.

If successful, pain will typically improve for a few hours until the medication wears off.

The next step involves burning the nerve, which should provide some pain relief for a few months until the nerve regrows. Because this doesn't affect the disease process itself, only the sensation, any instability, stiffness, or movement symptoms will stay and may even get worse unless other actions are taken.

There is no way to burn nerves to ease pain from spinal stenosis, but inflamed nerves in these conditions may respond to a mix of steroids and numbing medication. Your physician may prescribe an MRI as a way to plan these injections. An EMG might also come into play, used to figure out if existing nerves are experiencing active damage and inflammation. During the injection, your pain specialist may use fluoroscopy or ultrasound guidance to place the medication precisely at the nerve transmitting pain.

SHOULD I PLAN FOR INPATIENT REHABILITATION (IPR) AFTER SURGERY?

Typically, joint replacements and spinal decompressions or fusions don't require postoperative rehab. However, there are some situations where it's needed. One is when a surgery is very complex, such as multiple sections of the spine being fused or multiple joints being replaced at once or within weeks of each other. It's also recommended with significant other heart or lung problems, severe obesity, or if accompanied by neurologic problems like leg weakness and bowel or bladder changes. In these scenarios, IPR helps a person become safer and more independent when they're ultimately discharged home.

COMMON AND POTENTIAL COMPLICATIONS

Research backs the idea that simply knowing what to expect and what can go wrong with a major procedure increases a patient's satisfaction with the procedure, even if these complications occur. When it comes to orthopedic and spine surgery, these complications are important to understand. Parts of well-designed prehabilitation programs can reduce some of these risks.

For example, infection is a major potential risk after surgery. Any time the skin is punctured or cut, bacteria in the area can dive a little deeper and hide in the wound. For surgeries near the surface, this isn't a huge concern because topical and IV antibiotics during the surgery prevent bacteria from finding a home. If they evade the first line of defense, antibiotics after surgery can usually clear the infection.

In orthopedic and spine surgeries, this can be a very serious problem. Bacteria that nestle underneath an implanted joint (i.e., the "new knee") can hide and multiply for days and weeks before the patient or medical team realizes an infection is brewing.[118] Treating this infection starts with more IV antibiotics but can easily lead to a reoperation to "wash out" the area and possibly even replace the prosthetic. Or, in very rare worst case scenarios, it can lead to amputation of the limb. With a newly fused spine, bacteria can create an expanding self-contained mass of infection (an abscess) that may compress the spinal cord and cause nerve injury or paralysis.

The best thing patients can do to reduce these risks is to make the areas (their bodies) uninviting to bacteria. This includes removing bacteria's preferred food source—sugar—by tightly

---

[118] Rachid Rassir et al., "Is Obesity Associated with Short-Term Revision After Total Knee Arthroplasty? An Analysis of 121,819 Primary Procedures from the Dutch Arthroplasty Register," Knee 27, no. 6 (December 2020): 1899–1906, https://doi.org/10.1016/j.knee.2020.09.020.

controlling diabetes for patients with metabolic disease. Then, make sure that immune defenses can patrol the area by improving circulation with exercise during prehab. These strategies could also reduce the risk of blood clots.[119] Exercise and sleep improvements also directly improve immune system function.

Patients are at a high risk of blood clots due to the effects of orthopedic surgery itself, as well as from the reduced mobility after surgery. This is one reason your physical therapist might come off as a (welcome and playful) bully when they insist you bear weight on your new joint or spine fusion. Early mobility minimizes the risk of blood clots, and an intensive exercise program during prehab can make that early mobility after surgery even less painful. Your surgeon will also likely prescribe a blood thinner—aspirin, a medication like heparin, or newer oral anticoagulants—to reduce clotting function. If you're already on a blood thinner, that medication may take the place of aspirin or heparin. The approach varies based on the procedure, surgeon, and evolving research. The goal is to find the ideal balance between risk of clotting and bleeding.

Surgery revision due to infection has already been discussed and will make itself known within days or weeks of the first surgery, but a new surgery may also be required due to "hardware failure." This is when the implant loosens, breaks, or becomes dislocated. Research suggests that obesity increases the risk of revision after knee surgery.[120] This is likely the case for other joints and spine surgery for a few reasons.

---

119 Gemma Vilahur et al., "New Insights into the Role of Adipose Tissue in Thrombosis," *Cardiovascular Research* 113, no. 9 (July 2017): 1046–1054, https://doi.org/10.1093/cvr/cvx086.

120 Jonathan Thomas Evans et al., "Obesity and Revision Surgery, Mortality, and Patient-Reported Outcomes After Primary Knee Replacement Surgery in the National Joint Registry: A UK Cohort Study," *PLOS Medicine* 18, no. 7 (2021): 1–19, e1003704, https://doi.org/10.1371/journal.pmed.1003704; Akhil Katakam et al., "Obesity Increases Risk of Failure to Achieve the 1-Year PROMIS PF-10a Minimal Clinically Important Difference Following Total Joint Arthroplasty," *Journal of Arthroplasty* 36, no. 7 Supplement (July 2021): S184–S191, https://doi.org/10.1016/j.arth.2020.11.004.

First, things that make infection more likely—poor blood flow, high blood sugar, etc.—play a factor in overall healing. When circulation to the surgery area is poor, the body won't heal as well. The remaining bone doesn't heal well into and around the implanted joint or fusion rods and screws. This makes it more likely the hardware will loosen or break. Second, improper body mechanics due to other joint or spine issues can put high stress on the new hardware or turn it at an unexpected angle. High body weight can make this stress even greater.

Each of those factors ties back to why prehab is so important. Prehab can lower risks by strengthening muscles to take stress off the joint, improve body movement patterns, and control diabetes and other healing-related factors like poor sleep and nutrition.

ACTION POINTS

- Weight loss isn't the only prehabilitation goal before joint or spine surgery. Some surgeons do have strict maximum levels for body mass index (BMI), but a proper approach targets several areas. The most important are improving metabolic health, strengthening muscles, and correcting improper body movement patterns. These create a healthier environment around the area of surgery, improve the rate of healing, and reduce complication risks.
- Your team has several ways to control pain, but expect to work through the pain before and after surgery. Some pain control methods require time for full effect, and the goal will typically be to achieve "tolerable" pain.
- Assume you will begin physical therapy within one or two days after surgery.
- For simple fusions or joint replacements, assume you will

be discharged home within a few days of surgery. If you have significant disability before the operation or you've experienced surgical complications, this may require acute inpatient rehabilitation or subacute rehab (i.e., at a skilled nursing facility).

CHAPTER 4

CANCER TREATMENT PREHABILITATION

NEARLY 40 PERCENT OF PEOPLE WILL BE DIAGNOSED WITH cancer at some point in their lives.[121] The good news is that how we diagnose and treat cancer is constantly improving. Many diagnoses that used to stump medicine are now treatable and newly "curable" (remission). There's hope and plenty of real benefit to be had from understanding and preparing for the potentially long cancer treatment journey.

Prehabilitation is often critically important before cancer treatment. As we touched on earlier, physicians are beginning to widely accept that—in most cases—it's in a person's best interest to make time for prehab even if it may require delaying treatment. Where cancer differs from other diagnoses is that it may require both surgery and complementary treatment

---

[121] Melissa C. Hulvat, "Cancer Incidence and Trends," *Surgical Clinics of North America* 100, no. 3 (June 2020): 469–481, https://doi.org/10.1016/j.suc.2020.01.002; P. D. Sasieni et al., "What Is the Lifetime Risk of Developing Cancer?: The Effect of Adjusting for Multiple Primaries," *British Journal of Cancer* 105, no. 3 (2011): 460–465, https://doi.org/10.1038/bjc.2011.250.

like chemotherapy or radiation either before or after surgery. A single procedure presents challenges during recovery. The possibility of multiple treatments means that a prehabilitation program must really be up to the task and nimble enough to hit a constantly moving target.

On top of that, there are many examples when cancer is involved where a very worthy goal is stopping the disease in its tracks rather than pushing for a complete remission. Diagnoses like stage IV prostate cancer or breast cancer can be advanced enough where the idea of eliminating the cancer from the body entirely just isn't realistic. In those situations, you'll never reduce the cancer burden down to zero, but it may be possible to stop certain cancers from progressing. These people may always live with cancer, but that's the point—they're living. For them, cancer won't be the thing that kills them.

Cancer is the furthest thing from a diagnosis that always stays the same. It's one word used to summarize an extremely diverse group of diseases. Because cancer can be so diverse and unique to each person, our prehab and treatment strategies must be infinitely diverse. The goal might be to eradicate cancer from the body, or it might be to extend the quality portion of a person's life for six months. Both of those are admirable goals to have in their unique circumstances.

Treating cancer doesn't just have the potential to include multiple procedures. It also relies on a medical team made up of several disciplines. Knowing how this team operates and how different types of cancer behave can make you more prepared for prehab and beyond.

A REASON FOR HOPE

I was a first year pre-med student at the University of Pennsylvania in Philadelphia in 2012. While making breakfast in my cramped apartment "kitchen" that overlooked a poorly aging brick alley, I opened my laptop and read an incredible headline. For the first time that I'd ever seen, a small cohort of patients with acute leukemia were administered genetically engineered white blood cells and achieved *remission*. It sounded like something straight out of science fiction.

From my best recollection of the article that I can no longer find—my apologies—these patients received the therapy and had an unpleasant reaction with fever/chills and feeling generally unwell, and after making it through the worst of treatment... they felt better. Like, *better* better, and their subsequent tests supported it. As I progressed through medical education, the formal reports of larger-scale studies of CAR-T and other "*immunotherapies* (more on these later) corroborated these findings in specific, previously devastating cancer types like acute leukemia and melanoma.[122] Suddenly, the horizon opened to an entirely new, previously unexpected mechanism for treating cancer. I still get chills thinking about when I read that first article.

TREATMENT TEAM AND HELPFUL TERMINOLOGY

A patient with advanced cancer may see a few specialists, a surgical oncologist and a radiation oncologist, on top of sev-

---

122 Shannon L. Maude et al., "Chimeric Antigen Receptor T Cells for Sustained Remissions in Leukemia," *New England Journal of Medicine* 371, no. 16 (2014): 1507–1517, https://doi.org/10.1056/NEJMoa1407222; Sapna P. Patel et al., "Neoadjuvant–Adjuvant or Adjuvant-Only Pembrolizumab in Advanced Melanoma," *New England Journal of Medicine* 388, no. 9 (2023): 813–823, https://doi.org/10.1056/NEJMoa2211437.

eral other non-cancer-specific physicians. Most patients realize cancer treatments come with side effects, but the extent of these isn't quite as universally known. In comprehensive cancer treatment centers, a physiatrist or other rehab specialist will ideally be involved to lead prehab and postoperative rehab.

MEDICAL ONCOLOGISTS

Medical oncologists are specialists in the treatment of cancer who prescribe chemotherapy, immunotherapy, and other whole-body treatments. They work closely with other subspecialist oncologists and primary care doctors to develop a comprehensive cancer treatment plan. Medical oncologists use many tests to diagnose cancer and then recommend a plan based on the cancer's type, stage, and the patient's overall health.

These specialists treat a wide range of cancer types, including but not limited to blood cancers, lung cancer, breast cancer, and gastrointestinal cancers. They may also recommend palliative care designed to relieve cancer-related symptoms and improve quality of life.

SURGICAL ONCOLOGISTS

Surgical oncologists are specialists in the surgical treatment of cancer. Broadly, they perform various types of cancer surgeries, including tumor and lymph node removal and reconstructive surgeries. Surgical oncologists work with other oncologists to develop a treatment plan that may include surgery as the main treatment, preceded or followed by radiation or chemotherapy.

A patient may receive chemotherapy or immunotherapy or radiation before surgery in order to shrink the tumors in "neoadjuvant" treatments. These specialists may also perform biopsies to diagnose cancer and determine the cancer stage. Surgical oncologists are typically most involved with treatment in early-stage cancer that is localized and can be removed surgically.

RADIATION ONCOLOGISTS

Radiation oncologists specialize in the use of radiation therapy to treat cancer. They work with other oncologists to develop a total treatment plan that may include radiation therapy as the mainstay or in combination with surgery or chemotherapy. Radiation oncologists use beams of high-energy radiation to destroy cancer cells, and they work closely with physicists and dosimetrists (a specialty within nuclear medicine) to calculate the appropriate dosage and plan the radiation treatment.

Radiation oncologists treat various cancer types, including brain, prostate, and breast cancers. Their work is often most appropriate for patients with cancer that is localized or has spread to a limited area that can be treated with radiation.

DIETICIANS AND NUTRITIONISTS

These professionals play a critical role in the care of patients with cancer by providing nutritional counseling and support through treatment and rehabilitation. Cancer and its treatments can impact a person's appetite, nutritional requirements, digestion, and ability to eat. These issues can affect overall health and well-being and the recovery process. Therefore, proper nutrition is essential for patients to help maintain strength, minimize treatment side effects, and improve quality of life.

Dieticians and nutritionists work with patients to assess their nutritional status and develop personalized nutrition plans based on their specific needs, preferences, and medical histories. They also offer advice on how to manage side effects of treatment such as nausea, vomiting, or diarrhea. In addition to providing nutrition counseling, dieticians and nutritionists work with other members of the healthcare team, and they may also work closely with caregivers to provide guidance on how to prepare meals that meet the patients' nutritional needs.

PHYSICAL AND OCCUPATIONAL THERAPISTS

These therapists play an important role in both cancer pre-habilitation and rehabilitation by helping patients prevent and manage the physical effects of cancer and its treatments. Physical therapists design treatments to improve strength, flexibility, mobility, and endurance. This might involve therapies to improve range of motion, balance, and coordination, as well as ways to manage pain and swelling. Physical therapy can also help patients address the side effects of cancer, such as fatigue, weakness, and pain in joints, bones, and nerves. The therapy team anticipates these side effects and designs prehab programs that will directly reduce their negative impact and compensate for negative effects that might develop.

On the other hand, occupational therapy focuses on helping patients regain independence in their daily activities through new and modified ways to perform tasks like dressing, grooming, and cooking. These therapists also deal with issues related to cognitive and emotional functioning. For example, nerve pain caused by chemotherapy can impact balance and dexterity, both of which make previously simple tasks like buttoning a shirt or shaving more difficult to perform.

Occupational therapy can also help patients deal with the challenges of returning to work or other activities after treatment. The cancer rehab team works together to personalize physical and occupational therapies most suited to the needs of individual patients with cancer. This can be based on factors like the type of cancer, stage of the disease, and patient's overall health and fitness level.

CANCER PHYSIATRIST

A cancer physiatrist is a specialized version of a physical medicine and rehabilitation doctor (physiatrist) who specifically deals with cancer. This doctor prescribes treatments to improve how a patient functions before, during, and after cancer treatment. They work with the rest of the team to diagnose and treat conditions like frailty, nerve and other pain, lymphedema (swelling of legs or arms), and others to promote best quality of life after a cancer diagnosis.

RESPIRATORY THERAPISTS

Respiratory therapists play a very important role in cancer care for patients presently or likely to experience breathing difficulties after treatment. Respiratory therapists may also work with patients before surgery to strengthen breathing muscles and treat patients after surgery to regain lung function and prevent complications like pneumonia or atelectasis (lung collapse).

Radiation therapy to the chest and certain chemotherapy drugs can damage the lungs or surrounding respiratory tissues, which may cause shortness of breath and other symptoms. Respiratory therapists can help patients manage these symptoms through techniques like breathing exercises, oxygen therapy, or nebulizer treatments.

PSYCHOLOGISTS AND PSYCHIATRISTS

Psychologists, psychiatrists, and other mental health specialists are often involved in cancer treatment. Cancer comes with a heavy emotional burden on patients, especially for those who already have symptoms of depression and anxiety, or after someone receives a terminal diagnosis. Cancer treatments involving the brain might further impact mood. Considering all these factors, most patients with cancer would benefit from (at least) screening sessions with a mental health specialist. Depression and anxiety can have a negative impact on treatment outcomes and quality of life during survivorship, so treating them is a priority.

PALLIATIVE CARE

Palliative care specialists are team members involved in the well-being of patients who typically have severe, chronic, or terminal illnesses. They are specially trained to guide meaningful and self-reflective conversations with patients and their families regarding goals of care and long-term wishes.

These specialists work with psychiatrists and other mental health specialists to reduce pain, anxiety, or depression during treatment. The palliative care team helps coordinate caregiver support resources, a patient's transition to hospice care, and end-of-life care.

CANCER TERMINOLOGY AND TYPES

Maybe you've heard different terms used to describe cancer without understanding exactly what they mean or how they differ from one another. Carcinoma, sarcoma, melanoma, lymphoma, and leukemia are all types of cancers, but they arise from different tissues and have their own characteristics.

Carcinoma is a cancer that starts in the cells that make up the skin or the lining of organs. This could be the liver, lungs, or intestines. It is the most common "family" of cancer and can be further broken down into subtypes based on the specific cells affected.

Sarcomas are cancers that begin in connective tissues like bones, muscles, and cartilage. Relative to other types of cancer, sarcoma is rarer and can be divided into subtypes based on the type of tissue affected. For example, osteosarcoma is bone cancer and chondrosarcoma involves cartilage.

Melanoma is a specific type of skin cancer that comes from the pigment-producing cells called melanocytes. It is traditionally the most dangerous form of skin cancer and is less directly related to sun exposure over a person's lifetime. This type of cancer tends to metastasize, or spread, to other parts of the body.

Lymphoma is a cancer that affects the lymphatic system, which is the network of vessels and organs that help fight infection and disease. It may develop in any lymphoid tissue like the spleen, lymph nodes, and bone marrow.

Leukemia is a cancer that starts in the blood-forming cells, particularly the bone marrow. This results in the body producing too many abnormal white blood cells. It can be further classified into subtypes based on the type of white blood cell affected, such as "myeloid" or "lymphoid." The subtype lymphoid sounds close to lymphoma, but it actually describes blood cancers that come from the white blood cell family called lymphocytes.

Treatment for different types of cancer may vary depending on many factors, such as stage and location of the cancer, the patient's age and health status, and the aggressiveness of the cancer. Some common treatments include surgery, radiation therapy, chemotherapy, targeted therapy, and immunotherapy.

As we will detail later, surgery is often the first treatment choice for cancers that haven't spread to multiple areas, such as carcinoma or sarcoma *in situ* (meaning it hasn't spread). Surgery involves the removal of cancerous tissue and often precedes other treatments such as radiation or chemotherapy. Radiation is often used along with surgery, especially when the cancer is difficult to remove completely. It can also be used as the primary treatment for certain types of cancer, such as lymphoma.

Chemotherapy involves the use of drugs that target rapidly dividing cells, like cancer cells. It may be used alone or in combination with other treatments, such as surgery or radiation therapy. Chemotherapy is often the primary treatment for cancers that are inherent to an entire bodily system, like leukemia or lymphoma, or for cancers that have metastasized.

Targeted therapy is a specific kind of chemotherapy that targets the cancer cells' unique features, such as proteins or genes. It may be used alone or in combination with other treatments. One of the earliest target therapies was a drug called imatinib (Gleevec). Drug scientists developed this drug based on knowledge of the exact shape of the mutated protein that causes chronic myeloid leukemia.

As described earlier, immunotherapy uses the patient's immune system to fight cancer by boosting the immune response and training it to focus on specific markers on cancer cells. It is often used to treat advanced cancers, such as melanoma or lymphoma.

CARE OVERVIEW

A cancer diagnosis typically occurs through one of two routes: positive tests ordered because of symptoms and screening tests that are routinely ordered without symptoms. This section lays out the steps of a general cancer treatment process and the medical professionals involved using a (fictional) case study.

EXAMPLE CASE

A seventy-one-year-old male who has smoked one pack of cigarettes daily for most of his life has been unintentionally losing weight and has developed a chronic cough with mucus. When the mucus becomes streaked with blood, he speaks with his PCP. The PCP orders tests that identify lung cancer and recommends he see an oncologist.

This is where care becomes split between multiple specialists. Our patient visits a medical oncologist, surgical oncologist, and, potentially, a radiation oncologist. He should also visit a prehabilitation specialist who will work with the other oncology specialists and design a plan to fit within the time before treatment begins. This plan will likely involve meeting with physical and occupational therapists, and—given his weight loss—a nutritionist/dietician. The nutritionist will give recommendations for achieving the target weight and nutritional status. Since our patient is about to start treatment for lung cancer and may have other undiagnosed lung diseases, a respiratory therapist will provide important breathing therapies to prepare breathing muscles for chest radiation and/or surgery.

After this planning and prehab period, the patient will receive treatment involving a combination of chemotherapy, radiation therapy, and surgery. He will first receive neoadjuvant chemotherapy before surgery to shrink the tumor and improve the likelihood of removing as much of the cancer as possible with surgery.

Once all treatments are completed or there is a planned period of approximately three weeks between treatments, the patient may transfer to inpatient rehabilitation under certain conditions. Generally, to qualify for inpatient rehab, he will need to tolerate and benefit from three hours per day of a combination of physical, occupational, or speech therapy and have a situation complex enough to require active management from a physician. This may include adjusting diabetes medication, treating swallowing problems with specialty diets or tube feeding, and treating bowel or bladder problems requiring medications and retraining. If these conditions aren't met, a skilled nursing or subacute rehabilitation facility provides less intense daily therapies. There's a chance our patient could receive these treatments as an outpatient and not need inpatient rehab. In that case, he could also continue targeted outpatient therapies to maintain the gains achieved during prehab.

Moving forward, the patient will likely have ongoing follow-up visits with the different oncology subspecialists for maintenance therapy, monitoring, or additional courses of major therapy. He will continue to follow up with the prehab physician, or if prehab isn't completed, a dedicated cancer physiatrist can manage symptoms and side effects of treatment. These might be nerve pain from chemotherapy, nerve damage from radiation, or edema from surgery, for example.

One potential step is consultation with the palliative care team to assist in goals of care (GOC) planning. This happens regardless of whether the prognosis is favorable or poor. If his cancer is considered terminal, the palliative care team transitions the plan to "comfort measures," ensures care corresponds with his wishes, and avoids unwanted treatments.

PREHABILITATION PILLARS: CANCER TREATMENT

Prehab for cancer involves pulling all the levers at our disposal. All of the pillars apply here because the biology of cancer and chemoradiation chip away at each system. For example, patients with advanced cancer typically experience *cachexia*, a condition of muscle wasting, frailty, and fatigue.[123] The root cause is a complex relationship between inflammation that suppresses appetite while often increasing metabolic demand. The body is in an energy deficit, which leads to burning muscle for energy.

This state contrasts with one of the most common risk factors for developing cancer or suffering a recurrence: obesity. Some research suggests obesity is the second most preventable/"modifiable" influence on the development of cancer—surpassed only by smoking.[124] This is due to fat tissue releasing different hormones that raise inflammation, promote blood vessel growth, increase growth factors, and have other effects. On top of this, certain behaviors like inactivity and consuming high-calorie and processed foods promote both obesity and cancer development. Most cancers are associated with obesity or metabolic syndrome to some degree, but some of the most closely linked are breast, endometrial, ovarian, colorectal, pancreatic, and liver cancers. Liver cancer risk is more closely tied to fatty liver disease that leads to inflammation and cirrhosis.

This is not a conversation about how patients with obesity

---

[123] Roberta Sartori et al., "Perturbed BMP Signaling and Denervation Promote Muscle Wasting in Cancer Cachexia," *Science Translational Medicine* 13, no. 605 (2021): eaay9592, https://doi.org/10.1126/scitranslmed.aay9592.

[124] Giovanni De Pergola and Franco Silvestris, "Obesity as a Major Risk Factor for Cancer," *Journal of Obesity* 2013, no. 1 (January 2013): 2, 291546, http://dx.doi.org/10.1155/2013/291546; Konstantinos I. Avgerinos et al., "Obesity and Cancer Risk: Emerging Biological Mechanisms and Perspective," *Metabolism* 92 (March 2019): 121–135, https://doi.org/10.1016/j.metabol.2018.11.001.

and metabolic disease are at fault for getting cancer. In fact, this stigma (discussed later) is unproductive, unnecessary, and, frankly, unfair for reasons discussed in greater depth in the next chapter. Instead, the main point is that several weeks of an intense and well-rounded prehabilitation program can lead to meaningful potential benefits. There isn't much research to prove that survival is more likely with prehab participation, but one study showed that prehab increases time after first treatment before cancer returns ("disease-free survival") in patients with colorectal cancer.[125] Despite this finding, prehab didn't provide a benefit for overall survival—patients who participated in prehab passed away at about the same time as those who didn't go through prehabilitation.

Any time spent free of cancer is a worthy and admirable goal. Prehab can help with effects of cancer and its treatments, including muscle wasting and fatigue, but it also has the potential to improve quality of life before, during, and after treatment.

EXERCISE

Cancer prehab exercise regimens with the most benefit in the shortest time often involve high-intensity interval training (HIIT).[126] As we discussed in Chapter 1, this training style involves bursts of vigorous exercise at maximal intensity for short durations (approximately one minute) mixed with low-intensity recovery periods. Intensity is relative, so for someone

---

[125] Maude Trépanier et al., "Improved Disease-Free Survival After Prehabilitation for Colorectal Cancer Surgery," *Annals of Surgery* 270, no. 3 (September 2019): 493–501, https://doi.org/10.1097/SLA.0000000000003465.

[126] Stefano Palma et al., "High-Intensity Interval Training in the Prehabilitation of Cancer Patients—A Systematic Review and Meta-Analysis," *Supportive Care in Cancer* 29, no. 4 (2021): 1781–1794, https://doi.org/10.1007/s00520-020-05834-x.

who hasn't exercised in decades, it's perfectly reasonable that thirty seconds of "light" jogging could take their full effort. If this is part of your prehabilitation program, expect close oversight at first for safety reasons.

HIIT can greatly improve peak aerobic capacity ("cardio") in relatively short periods, but a well-designed exercise regimen will also include resistance training. This is done to build "insurance-policy" muscle in case of loss later and to increase resilience to injury. In general, there are a few weight training modifications that are best for cancer prehab. One standard rule is to avoid resistance training in a limb that has a cancer metastasis. If there is a bony tumor in an arm or leg, lifting weights may stress that bone and put it at risk of "pathologic fracture" if enough force is involved. If a tumor is closer to the midline in an area that may still be stressed with compound (multi-joint exercises), your physiatrist or physical therapist may recommend blood-flow restriction training. As we discussed, BFR makes resistance training with light weight more effective. For patients with cancer, research confirms that BFR along with whey protein, the amino acid citrulline, and creatine supplements can significantly increase muscle mass and reduce fat in only four weeks.[127] Although available research also shows that short bursts of BFR aren't associated with risk of blood clots, the "hypercoagulable state" caused by many cancers means the decision to use BFR is a nuanced discussion of risks versus benefits.

Pelvic floor exercise is a crucial exercise type to include in prehab for prostate and other pelvic cancers. By participating in pelvic floor exercises before surgery, individuals may

---

[127] Savannah V. Wooten et al., "Prehabilitation Program Composed of Blood Flow Restriction Training and Sports Nutrition Improves Physical Functions in Abdominal Cancer Patients Awaiting Surgery," *European Journal of Surgical Oncology* 47, no. 11 (November 2021): 2952–2958, https://doi.org/10.1016/j.ejso.2021.05.038.

significantly increase their likelihood of maintaining bladder continence (being able to hold their urine) after cancer treatment.[128]

LIFESTYLE

If you currently smoke, the very best lifestyle intervention is to stop smoking. This lowers the risk of developing any lung diseases in the future but also helps improve the effectiveness of exercise and nutritional interventions. Certain life events can make major habit changes more likely to "stick," and receiving a cancer diagnosis is likely one of those events. Because there is a chance of short-term symptoms like increased phlegm or coughing, stopping smoking as soon as possible will ensure these symptoms pass by the end of the prehab period. Certain medications like bupropion, nicotine, and varenicline may help reduce the urge to smoke while quitting.

Nutritional supplements may add value in all prehab programs, but some are especially beneficial when faced with certain cancers that may increase the need for certain vitamins, minerals, and nutrients. For instance, patients with colorectal cancer are often anemic because the tumors slowly bleed into the GI tract, which gets carried out with stool. This causes patients to often have low iron levels. Supplements like creatine monohydrate and whey protein may be beneficial for building and maintaining muscle and preventing overtraining from exercise.

It's worth noting that new research suggests anti-inflammatory supplement combinations may reduce the

---

128 C. Treanor et al., "An International Review and Meta-Analysis of Prehabilitation Compared to Usual Care for Cancer Patients," *Journal of Cancer Survivorship* 12, no. 1 (2018): 64–73, https://doi.org/10.1007/s11764-017-0645-9.

inflammatory aspect of muscle wasting and cachexia in advanced cancers.[129] Combining supplements like fish oil with anti-inflammatory medications like celecoxib, traditional appetite stimulants like mirtazapine, and caloric supplements can have a greater-than-normal benefit on someone experiencing rapid weight loss.

Weight management in cancer prehab takes on a very deliberate strategy. Unlike prehab for other interventions like bariatric, orthopedic, and spine surgery, the approach to weight in cancer prehab is more similar to the approach for high-risk pregnancy. Instead of pushing for weight loss (for metabolic health) or weight gain (for "reserve" building), prehab for cancer treatment usually focuses on weight maintenance and optimizing body composition. This means we don't necessarily want to change the number on the scale too much, but we are trying to carefully build muscle while burning fat even if it means being more gradual. Research suggests that weight gain and weight (muscle) loss may promote worse outcomes from cancer treatment.[130] Good nutrition via monitoring total calories and prioritizing protein may keep the scale steady while building muscle and burning some excess fat.

---

129 Tora S. Solheim et al., "Non-Steroidal Anti-Inflammatory Treatment in Cancer Cachexia: A Systematic Review," *Acta Oncologica* 52, no. 1 (2013): 6–17, https://doi.org/10.3109/02841 86X.2012.724536.

130 Candyce H. Kroenke et al., "Weight, Weight Gain, and Survival After Breast Cancer Diagnosis," *Journal of Clinical Oncology* 23, no. 7 (2005): 1370–1378, https://doi.org/10.1200/ JCO.2005.01.079; Kenneth C. Fearon et al., "Definition of Cancer Cachexia: Effect of Weight Loss, Reduced Food Intake, and Systemic Inflammation on Functional Status and Prognosis," *American Journal of Clinical Nutrition* 83, no. 6 (June 2006): 1345–1350, https:// doi.org/10.1093/ajcn/83.6.1345.

NEUROPSYCHIATRIC

This pillar is very important in cancer prehabilitation. In the realm of mood disorders, depression and adjustment disorders are common after receiving a new diagnosis of cancer. Worse, some cancers like lung, liver, and others associated with obesity often come with additional feelings of guilt and stigma. This can be due to their ties with behaviors like smoking, drinking, and overeating, even for patients who don't do these things to excess.

Mood disorders may impact motivation, sleep, and other important factors for maximizing participation in prehab, cancer treatments, and post-treatment monitoring. Grief counselors, psychiatrists, psychologists, and other mental health specialists have important roles in most patients' cancer care.

During a cancer battle, brain chemistry may change either from the mental distress, as a side effect of treatments, or from other factors like systemic inflammation.[131] Insomnia is a large burden for many patients with cancer. As we've discussed, sleep is underappreciated but a crucial piece of good health. Enough quality sleep causes nearly every bodily process to function optimally—recovery from exercise, blood sugar regulation, mood support, pain tolerance, and others. In fact, poor sleep over long periods may be a risk factor for cancer development itself.[132]

Undertreating insomnia while battling cancer can negatively impact the journey. Proper treatment may involve medications that can treat two symptoms. For example, patients with nerve

---

[131] Daniel C. McFarland et al., "Cancer-Related Inflammation and Depressive Symptoms: Systematic Review and Meta-Analysis," *Cancer* 128, no. 13 (2022): 2504–2519, https://doi.org/10.1002/cncr.34193.

[132] Sayato Fukui et al., "Both Increased and Decreased Sleep Duration over Time Are Associated with Subsequent Cancer Development," *Sleep and Breathing* 26, no. 4 (2022): 2035–2043, https://doi.org/10.1007/s11325-021-02517-7; D. Kobayashi and T. Shimbo, "Longitudinal Sleep Duration and Subsequent Development of Cancer in the Japanese Population," *Neoplasma* 67, no. 5 (2020): 1182–1190, https://doi.org/10.4149/neo_2020_200219N154.

pain may benefit from a medication like amitriptyline or doxepin at bedtime. Others who have poor appetite and mood may instead benefit from a medication like mirtazapine.

Cancer-related fatigue is another big issue, particularly because it has many causal factors and can overlap with cachexia—muscle wasting/weight loss overall. When it comes to fatigue, depression and "adjustment disorder" are big factors, as is the inflammatory state caused by the cancer itself. Treatment options include supplements and, as implied early, anti-inflammatories like celecoxib. Poor nutrition and poor sleep worsen cancer-related fatigue and everything that contributes to it. Fatigue can become so severe that patients can't engage in *any* physical activity, so addressing it early is critically important.

Finally, pain control in cancer therapy extends beyond the typical joint and back pain programs that generally avoid opioids. For many cancer treatment courses, patients should anticipate a combination of short- and long-acting opioids to dull the gnawing, aching pain that certain cancers bring. In some cases, fully participating in physical therapy might require opioids to prevent being limited by pain and losing out on potential therapeutic benefit.

Pain management for cancer care involves other unique measures, particularly for pain from tumors within bones. These may require radiation therapy to suppress tumor growth and lower local inflammation. Medications like bisphosphonates (traditionally used in osteoporosis) that reduce bone breakdown are another option. Nasal spray formulations of medications like calcitonin can also slow the breakdown of bone and the related pain.

The prehab pillars lead us into how best to set expectations during cancer treatment.

EXPECTATION MANAGEMENT

There are a few important points to manage expectations of cancer prehabilitation. First, consider involving the palliative care team *early* in treatment. Their involvement isn't just for end-of-life care, and they can help patients and their families navigate transitions in care like going from active treatment to passively monitoring for disease recurrence. They also provide resources such as information on support groups and peer networks, and their expertise includes guiding patients through difficult decisions. Often, individuals request palliative care's involvement long after they may have benefited from their guidance.

Medicine is at a stage of being able to extract additional days, weeks, and months of life from difficult treatments. An objective and sensitive professional can help patients identify what is truly important to them, potentially avoiding a trade-off of meaningful quality of life for a small increase in quantity of life.

Second, don't overlook the exhausting demand of cancer fatigue and chronic pain. When participating in intensive prehab or inpatient rehab, therapy may require a daily "summoning of strength" when every fiber is telling you to rest. Even when there is enough rest and recovery in off periods, perseverance will feel like a monumental feat at times. Acknowledge this, but don't let it stop you. Dig deep, and power through. Extract the maximal benefit from these therapies when able. Know yourself, and learn to tell the difference between when you *wish* you could rest versus when you actually *must* rest. Knowing when you can push through will help you maximize benefits, and it may make your rest periods all the more restful.

DELAY SURGERY REQUIREMENT

In other chapters, the "Delay Surgery" sections are typically intended to give patients ways to buy some time before surgery when it's their best and, eventually, only option. For cancer-related surgeries, this type of delay requires very important circumstances because delay can give cancer an opportunity to grow or spread. However, surgical oncologists are becoming increasingly supportive of short-term delays for prehabilitation in specific circumstances.[133] For locally spreading cancers, neoadjuvant chemotherapy can also shrink the tumor's reach.

---

[133] Maud T. A. Strous et al., "Impact of Therapeutic Delay in Colorectal Cancer on Overall Survival and Cancer Recurrence—Is There a Safe Timeframe for Prehabilitation?," *European Journal of Surgical Oncology* 45, no. 12 (December 2019): 2295–2301, https://doi.org/10.1016/j.ejso.2019.07.009; Anna Shukla et al., "Attitudes and Perceptions to Prehabilitation in Lung Cancer," *Integrative Cancer Therapies* 19 (2020): 1534735420924466, https://doi.org/10.1177/1534735420924466.

SHOULD I PLAN FOR INPATIENT REHABILITATION?

Inpatient rehabilitation or a skilled nursing facility might be a stop along the way at a few different points during cancer treatment. Typically, prehab alone isn't a strong enough reason for insurance to cover inpatient rehab *before* any other therapy has occurred. However, some unfortunate situations may have this as a silver lining. For example, one patient with whom I worked had recently been diagnosed with ovarian cancer. In order to have a chest port (an access point to infuse chemotherapy without risking damage to small veins in the arms) placed, she had to briefly stop taking blood-thinning medications. She formed a blood clot that traveled to her brain as an "embolic" stroke. This stroke caused new weakness and some difficulty finding her words. She hadn't begun any treatment for her cancer, but because of her stroke, she qualified for inpatient rehabilitation, which effectively became a prehab program as well. Other comorbidities may similarly warrant rehab prior to cancer therapy, and with some guidance, therapy plans can incorporate prehab-specific goals like resistance and balance training, among others.

After treatment, acute inpatient rehab (at least three hours of daily therapies) or subacute inpatient rehab (less than three hours of daily therapy) may occur after the first surgical treatment and chemotherapy. Individuals have already undergone a major intervention that resulted in needing help regaining certain functions. Patients with limited prognoses or even those who don't wish to participate in ongoing cancer treatments may still benefit from rehab to improve their function and quality of life. The time invested in rehab should be weighed against the time remaining.

COMMON AND POTENTIAL COMPLICATIONS

Most of us know someone who has undergone cancer treatments. Some side effects and complications are obvious—hair loss, weight loss, and surgical recovery. Others are less obvious and, in many cases, can be far more disruptive to quality of life.

Peripheral neuropathy is a general term for damage to the nerves outside of the brain or spinal cord. This is a common side effect of certain chemotherapy drugs. Typical symptoms include numbness, tingling, burning, and altered sensations in the ends of the longest nerves—the tips of fingers and toes. As this progresses, the distribution is often referred to as "stocking-glove," as hands and feet are most affected. Three chemotherapy agents are most likely to cause peripheral neuropathy:

- Platinum-based: Carboplatin, cisplatin, and oxaliplatin. These are commonly used for "solid" cancers like lung, ovarian, bladder, and testicular cancer.
- Taxanes: Paclitaxel and docetaxel. These are prescribed for most solid cancers, including breast, prostate, lung, and ovarian cancer.
- Vinca alkaloids: Vinblastine and vincristine. These are commonly prescribed for types of leukemia or lymphoma and solid tumors.

Besides nerve pain, some chemotherapy agents can cause hearing loss, heart damage, and lung damage.

Plexopathy is a term for some injury of nerve plexuses, essentially a location where nerves that have come out of the spine (spinal nerves or roots) mix and match fibers within them to create the peripheral nerves that go to our muscles and provide sensations in limbs. Plexus usually refers to the brachial plexus and the lumbosacral plexus, which create the nerves that run into our arms and legs, respectively.

Nerves in the plexus are sensitive to injury because they have limited ability to move in response to traction and other forces. This is very relevant if they get caught in the crossfire of radiation therapy. The main theory of how radiation therapy harms plexuses is that the radiation causes the surrounding tissue to scar, which compresses and distorts the shape of the plexus.

Plexopathies that affect the arms are more likely to occur when treating cancers near the region between the neck and axilla (armpit) with radiation therapy. This applies to breast and lung cancer. Leg plexopathies are more likely to occur after radiation to the pelvis, such as when treating prostate, cervical, or endometrial cancer. Plexus injuries are more likely to occur with chemotherapies that are likely to injure nerves, like those listed above. Both types of plexopathies can result in numbness, muscle weakness, and pain.

Lymphedema is a side effect of any injury to the lymph nodes or lymphatic system. This most commonly occurs after surgical removal and radiation to the axillary lymph nodes when treating breast cancer. Treatment for gynecologic or prostate cancer may injure pelvic lymph nodes, resulting in lymphedema in the groin, legs, or lower abdomen. The most common effect is swelling of the affected area.

One last note is that cancer treatment, like most things in medicine, is about finding balance. The agents that kill cancer, like we've touched on, can also do harm to our bodies. For example, radiation can increase the risk for other cancers. Immunotherapy can potentially cause autoimmune conditions to develop.

This list of potential complications is not meant to be exhaustive, as a full list would require volumes to discuss, even if the conditions described are very rare. The point is that your team will discuss the unique benefits and risks of your treatment with you, but your ultimate decisions are personal to you and your loved ones.

PSYCHEDELICS IN END-OF-LIFE CARE

Psilocybin and other psychedelic medicines offer many patients suffering from depression quicker relief than what normally comes from SSRIs and psychotherapy. These medications offer special uses in cancer-related care for managing end-of-life anxiety.

Multiple studies have shown that a single session of psilocybin can significantly improve both state (the result of a transient event) and trait (underlying behavioral patterns of an individual) anxiety.[134] Psilocybin can reduce fear of death in patients with terminal illness, essentially allowing them to be mindful and present in their remaining days so they can spend meaningful time with family and friends.

Importantly, psilocybin and other psychedelic medications that likely offer similar benefits have few, if any, interactions with other medications and disease states. Even if they did, their effects come from a single dose instead of the standard daily dosing. As psychedelic medications are further studied, researchers, physicians, and patient advocates have an opportunity to lobby against the stigma and arguably irresponsible across-the-board legal restrictions.

---

[134] Chia-Ling Yu et al., "Psilocybin for End-of-Life Anxiety Symptoms: A Systematic Review and Meta-Analysis," *Psychiatry Investigation* 18, no. 10 (2021): 958–967, https://doi.org/10.30773/pi.2021.0209.

ACTION POINTS

- Cancer prehabilitation focuses on improving the function and health of systems that are most likely to be affected by cancer treatment. This includes breathing exercises for chest surgeries, building and maintaining lean muscle for upcoming chemotherapy that may lead to weight loss or surgeries that may affect eating, and balance exercises if neuropathy may occur.
- Lifestyle changes focus on building muscle with less concern about fat loss. The caloric restrictions needed for fat loss would risk muscle loss. Other lifestyle treatments include stopping smoking and alcohol consumption and nutritional supplements to address nutrient deficiencies.
- Several types of cancer are closely tied to obesity and metabolic disease. This association means that improving metabolic health is one potent way to lower cancer risk.
- "Neuropsych" interventions often focus on mood disorders like depression or illness-related anxiety. This makes sure patients have the energy and focus for the medical fight at hand. If the prognosis turns terminal, new approaches with psychedelic-assisted psychotherapy can offer interested patients a "spiritual" approach to come to terms with the next stage of life.

CHAPTER 5

BARIATRIC SURGERY PREHABILITATION

IT IS ALL TOO COMMON FOR A PERSON TO FEEL LIKE HAVING overweight or obesity (the preferred terminology over "being obese") is their fault. The stigma that comes with these conditions has worked its way into mainstream culture and can make it seem like everything leading up to that diagnosis was a series of poor, avoidable choices.

This stigma isn't accurate or grounded in reality. There is much more involved that leads to someone developing obesity than just bad choices. Not only will this chapter detail the main factors that lead to obesity in the scope of effective prehabilitation, but it will point out healthy changes to combat them.

On the other hand, bariatric surgery is a powerful tool that must be taken seriously. It is far from a silver bullet or quick fix for those aiming to lose weight fast because surgery requires a lot of hard work and preparation. Surgery also creates anatomical changes that can last throughout the patient's life and is far more complicated than flipping a switch and losing weight.

Being mindful of things like the postoperative supplement regimen and minor risk of complications is crucial before choosing surgery. Like most major interventions, there will be a long road ahead. How you prepare for that road makes a difference.

Bariatric surgery prehab is unique in its length, members of the medical team involved, and scope of its risk factors. For example, while cancer prehab is often around four to six weeks in length, bariatric surgery prehab may last six to twelve months. While most of the team members for cancer prehab are oncologists or palliative care specialists and orthopedic prehab mostly involves orthopedists and pain management, bariatric surgery prehab involves a (often mandatory) group of specialists including psychologists, nutritionists, and others.

These unique features are all related to the procedure's nature—bariatric surgery is major elective surgery that permanently alters gastrointestinal (stomach and intestines) and hormonal systems. An orthopedic surgeon can fix poor outcomes of a joint implant by putting in another. Cancer treatment aims to return a patient as close to their original, pre-cancer health as possible. When successful, entirely elective bariatric surgery permanently alters the way patients' bodies process food and regulate energy and appetite.

However, the decision often doesn't exactly feel "elective" when it comes to bariatric surgery. These individuals have typically experienced a lifetime of struggling with their weight because *biology* dealt them a difficult set of cards. Obesity has deep genetic roots within genes that regulate appetite, fat and carbohydrate utilization, and energy production. For every person who can seemingly eat whatever they like without gaining a pound, the opposite is true for a person who appears to gain weight no matter *what* they eat. If the former person got "lucky" for their physiology, then it's only fair to remove guilt and stigma from the latter person for their "unlucky" situation. Even this description oversimplifies the complex relationship between our brains' appetite regulation, mitochondrial energy production, and muscle insulin sensitivity within a world where high-calorie food is becoming cheaper and easier to access.

Individuals with obesity are struggling with a chronic disease in the same way that someone with poor eyesight, cystic fibrosis, or Huntington's disease lacks complete influence over their health outcomes. Lifestyle factors can impact the chronic disease of obesity, but in most cases patients need sustainable therapy with medications or surgery to achieve "remission." Recognizing the struggle and removing the blame are the first steps we must take. From there, it can be helpful to understand exactly what we're talking about.

TREATMENT TEAM AND SURGERY TYPES

Even without including a dedicated prehabilitation team, the group of specialists involved in preparation for bariatric surgery looks very similar to a comprehensive prehab team. The following roster describes the standard treatment team for a Bariatric Surgery Center of Excellence—an accredited program that meets elevated standards.

SURGICAL AND MEDICAL WEIGHT LOSS TEAM

The bariatric surgeon evaluates how appropriate individuals are for surgery and presents different treatment options based on risks and benefits. If the patient is designated a surgical candidate, the surgery team (surgeon and PA/NP) will recommend further evaluation with the rest of the team.

Obesity medicine physicians are the nonsurgical weight

management specialists. Often, these specialists work together with the surgical team to reduce a patient's risk for surgery. This is often done by prescribing anti-obesity medications, nutrition and exercise recommendations, and, in some cases, fasting/meal replacement strategies.

SLEEP MEDICINE

Sleep specialists are "conditionally necessary" team members. With worsening obesity (higher BMI), the risk for obstructive sleep apnea (OSA) increases steadily. OSA itself worsens risk for high blood pressure, diabetes, heart attack, stroke, and pain. Additionally, untreated OSA may also raise the risk for complications during surgery.

BEHAVIORAL HEALTH

Psychologists or other mental health specialists are involved early in the surgical qualification period. They assess the risk of surgical stress, restrictive diet, and recovery period in causing or worsening psychiatric disorders like depression, anxiety, and addiction. Part of this evaluation includes determining the strength of a patient's support network—there need to be people a patient can rely on for help during recovery.

NUTRITIONAL TEAM

Registered dieticians play a similar role in bariatric surgery as they do in other well-rounded prehab programs. For patients awaiting surgery, especially those about to go through "malabsorptive" procedures like gastric bypass, the dietician plays a critical role in personalizing a meal plan. This must be sustainable and meet certain important metrics like total protein and vitamin and mineral content.

PAIN MANAGEMENT AND PHYSICAL MEDICINE

Pain management physicians and physiatrists are not usually formally included in the treatment team for bariatric surgery. However, they can play an invaluable role. Some patients use the outcomes of bariatric surgery, like weight loss and diabetes control, to qualify for orthopedic or spine surgeries. This becomes a chicken-and-egg situation where an individual with obesity needs weight loss to qualify for orthopedic surgery but struggles to lose weight due to pain limiting their exercise participation.

These are prime situations in which a physiatrist may treat pain and design personalized exercise plans and physical therapy to increase activity participation. Some of these doctors have additional specialized training in pain management such as advanced epidural procedures, ultrasound-guided nerve blocks, and other technical interventions. Note: pain management physicians may instead have trained as anesthesiologists prior to pain management fellowship.

Similar to finding the right treatment team, the choice of specific surgical procedure significantly impacts surgical outcomes and risk. Each intervention comes with its own benefits, risks, and type of patients who will be most appropriate. Surgeons are constantly studying different techniques for safer and more effective procedures. This list is meant to be broadly descriptive but not fully exhaustive.

Gastric Banding (Lap-Band™)

This is a procedure in which a literal band is placed around the stomach to reduce its volume for storing food. It is adjustable and removable but offers the lowest expected "excess body weight" loss of 30 to 50 percent. Metabolic benefits are directly due to weight loss alone, not any hormonal changes that come directly from surgery.

Vertical Sleeve Gastrectomy (VSG or the "Gastric Sleeve")

A gastric sleeve is a procedure in which the surgeon removes a section of the stomach. This creates a vertical, sleeve-shaped stomach. Removing tissue makes the stomach release less hunger hormones, leading to better appetite control. Patients can expect to lose 50 to 70 percent of their excess body weight.

Malabsorptive Procedures

This group includes the remaining types of bariatric surgeries. These include, but are not limited to, the Roux-en-Y gastric bypass, the biliopancreatic diversion with duodenal switch, and the loop duodenal switch. These are more technically challenging than the other procedures and involve rerouting the path food takes from the stomach and through the intestine. This reduces the amount of intestine that can absorb eaten calories. These procedures also reduce the size of the stomach. Together, they are both restrictive (stomach size) and malabsorptive (intestinal absorption). This combination leads to fewer calories eaten and less ability to absorb them.

In these, risks of malnutrition and deficiencies are highest, but weight loss is also highest. These may result in anywhere from 60 to 80 percent loss of excess body weight and will change the levels of circulating hormones, potentially fixing diabetes faster than weight loss alone.

CARE OVERVIEW

Care before, during, and after bariatric surgery follows a general sequence that looks something like this. Traditionally, lifestyle modifications and non-specialist care come first during meetings with a primary care physician. These include guidance on lifestyle changes for weight loss or participation in nonmedical, commercial weight loss programs.

The education period before surgery is usually managed by a medical weight loss specialist or subject-specific expert for the discussion at hand (nutritionist for diet, exercise physiologist or physical therapist for exercise, etc.). This may occur at the same time as the surgical team evaluation period, and this portion of the process could last three months or longer. Some insurance plans may not have any waiting period for certain surgical candidates. This aspect is evolving to move away from mandated waiting periods, with some insurers/geographic areas evolving faster than others.

If it doesn't happen at the same time, this is followed by the surgical team consultation and screening. Patients will meet with this team—surgeon, nutritionist, and psychologist—at the very least. If the surgeon recommends surgery, a patient will then meet with the nutritionist and psychologist for evaluations.

The time immediately before surgery may involve certain final tests and recommendations designed for final preparations. Active smokers should stop smoking at least four weeks before surgery but, ideally, starting at the very first consultation. A brief liquid-only fasting period starts a day before the surgery, and anti-nausea medications are provided immediately before surgery.

Surgery is then followed by immediate postoperative care and a period where the diet consists of only liquids, vitamins, and proton pump inhibitors (to reduce stomach acid). Gradually, the diet progresses from liquids to limited, easy-to-digest solids and slowly back to the new standard diet—frequent small meals and supplements.

Following surgery and immediate recovery, care transitions to continuing long-term lifestyle changes. Depending on the surgery, nutritional supplements with very specific composition may be necessary. Exercise and diet prescriptions need to continue supporting fat loss while limiting the loss of muscle mass.

PREHABILITATION PILLARS: BARIATRIC SURGERY

The prehab pillars make up the basis of how patients will prepare for bariatric surgery. As with every other form of prehab covered in this book, they use a combination of exercise, lifestyle modifications, and neuropsychiatric interventions.

EXERCISE

Exercise leading up to bariatric surgery is built on the foundation of "Something is better than nothing." Any incremental or small increase in activity is a good thing. Many individuals with obesity and chronic pain find that aquatic therapy—combining the benefits of aerobic and light resistance training in a heated pool—provides a more comfortable environment to begin retraining their bodies. Pool therapies can be within shared sessions for the social benefits and accountability of group exercise. In fact, research has shown that group exercise of any type with peers at a similar exercise level improves outcomes.[135]

Individuals who are using exercise and prehab both for weight loss and to control metabolic disease may achieve greater success with combining different exercise styles. High-intensity interval training (HIIT) is a method that basically trains different metabolic/muscle fiber systems, mixing anaerobic sprints with aerobic endurance training. HIIT, by nature, is a level of intensity some may find overwhelming. However, individuals can mix and match variations of brief high-intensity periods and casual low-intensity recovery periods until they find a tolerable ratio of high to low. "High-intensity" is a relative term, so no one is expecting a "five-minute mile" pace on day one...or days two to sixty, for that matter.

Resistance (strength) training is the best way to build muscle, and it is highly effective with sets to failure of eight to twenty repetitions (reps). There are many different set and rep combinations, but generally, more reps (in the eight to twelve range) combines the benefits of targeting both muscle and strength adaptation. Broadly, many low-repetition sets with heavy weight are more effective for building strength but not as ideal for building muscle. Strength is important for functional independence and fall recovery, but muscle mass is a critical long-term factor for controlling diabetes and physical resilience to trauma like falls and motor vehicle accidents. The more muscle you have, the more places your body can store excess sugar when it spikes.

---

[135] Gregory G. Kolden et al., "A Pilot Study of Group Exercise Training (GET) for Women with Primary Breast Cancer: Feasibility and Health Benefits," *Psycho-Oncology* 11, no. 5 (September/October 2002): 447–456, https://doi.org/10.1002/pon.591; Gail Powell-Cope et al., "Perceived Benefits of Group Exercise Among Individuals with Peripheral Neuropathy," *Western Journal of Nursing Research* 36, no. 7 (2014): 855–874, https://doi.org/10.1177/0193945914523493.

Cross-training simply means combining different exercise styles. One more reason it leads to maximum benefit is that it offers the opportunity to work out for extra days during the week without the same risk of overtraining or working the *same* muscle the *same* way, day in and day out. Only training with weights or only running at the necessary intensity to maximize benefits in a four- to six-week period increases the risk of overtraining or getting injured, particularly for the previously exercise-naive person. Instead, if the same time is divided between aerobic training and resistance training with progressively increasing the difficulty, individuals will likely obtain the greatest health and, likely, weight loss benefits.

A head-to-head comparison of multiple exercise modalities found that aquatic therapy and resistance training may both independently provide the greatest benefits for pain reduction, quality of life, and limiting fear or avoidant behaviors related to pain.[136] These helped more than other types of exercise including aerobic, yoga, and pilates. As has been stressed throughout this book, however, the first and "best" type of exercise is whichever one you can perform *consistently*!

As noted in the Exercise pillar in Chapter 1, a typical pyramid-style resistance repetition/set scheme may offer some variety. For example, if you can complete ten repetitions of the leg press machine with one hundred pounds of resistance, start the first warm-up without any weight on the machine to get your muscles ready for the appropriate form. Follow this with a progressive warm-up such as:

---

[136] Joseph G. Wasser et al., "Exercise Benefits for Chronic Low Back Pain in Overweight and Obese Individuals," PM & R 9, no. 2 (February 2017): 181–192, https://doi.org/10.1016/j.pmrj.2016.06.019.

- Set 1: Twenty to thirty pounds for twelve to fifteen reps
- Set 2: Forty to fifty pounds for eight to ten reps
- Set 3: Seventy to eighty pounds for four to six reps
- Set 4 (optional): Ninety to ninety-five pounds for one to two reps

Rest for a few minutes between sets if your ultimate health goal is to build strength. If your goal is more aerobic benefit at the expense of strength gains, shorter rest between sets will work better. But don't perform *any* resistance exercises with any significant resistance if you are unsure of the proper form. If you feel like a certain exercise just doesn't feel right—stop. Remember to discuss this with your own personal medical team and adhere to safe exercise guidelines introduced in earlier chapters. Anyone with a known or suspected metabolic disease like diabetes, high blood pressure, kidney disease, or heart disease who isn't already exercising should consult their physician before starting an exercise program. For those already lightly exercising, a physician should give the green light before increasing the intensity. When an individual is at particularly high risk, this health review may involve specialized testing like a stress test, electrocardiogram (EKG), or echocardiography.

Again, you should absolutely consult your PCP prior to starting or increasing an exercise regimen. They will help determine your level of risk and which testing or risk-minimizing strategies might be necessary. This isn't just to make sure that you're immediately well enough to participate in exercise. Prescreening may also provide reassurance that if symptoms arise during exercise—shortness of breath and fast heart rate are common—they are normal responses and unlikely to be the start of something like a heart attack.

Blood-flow restriction training is an exercise style introduced earlier (see Chapter 1) that can help individuals resistance train despite physical limitations like arthritis, high BMI, and poor balance. One study looked at the energy expenditure ("burn") caused by adding BFR to standard aerobic training in individuals with obesity. Not only did this result in burning more calories, but the individuals in the study did not perceive the increased effort, despite actually working harder. This means that BFR isn't just used to work around physical limitations. It can be part of a more "complete" workout even with limited use.

LIFESTYLE

Exercise is not the strongest intervention to promote weight loss. Weight loss fundamentally requires consuming fewer calories than you use in a day, period. Factors like activity level, diet type, and medications can change the number of calories required, but ultimately consuming fewer calories is the only way to force the body to burn stored energy—fat and carbohydrates. Most weight loss medications work to suppress appetite, making it easier to eat fewer calories. Diet and fasting strategies work by allowing you to sustain a calorie deficit, *not* by sidestepping the requirement.

Luckily, you aren't limited to medications or iron willpower in order to take in fewer calories. Behavioral "nudges" may help you shave off calories here and there in your diet. These can add up to real weight loss over time. Incorporate some of the following tactics into your life:

- Swap sugar with natural sweeteners like stevia, monk fruit extract, or allulose or with artificial sweeteners like aspartame or sucralose. This is a hot-button topic, but for weight loss (and health related to it), the studies are clear: artificial sweeteners are objectively healthier than sugar.[137] If you can tolerate *no* sweetener, then this may be even better, but don't feel guilty about the occasional diet soda or Sweet'N Low or Splenda if it keeps you on track.

- Keep healthy snacks visible and easily accessible. This can help you make healthier snacking choices and avoid less healthy impulses when hunger strikes.
- Use smaller plates and bowls. This can help control portion sizes and reduce calorie intake without feeling deprived.
- Drink water before meals. This helps you feel fuller and reduces the amount of food you consume during meals.
- Keep unhealthy foods out of sight. If you can't remove them from the grocery list, this can help you avoid temptation and make healthier food choices later at home.
- Plan your meals ahead of time, and make enough for leftovers. This can lead to healthier choices and less impulsive decisions when you've got limited options later.
- Read food labels. Knowing what you're eating helps you make more informed choices. It also becomes easier to avoid highly processed or high-sugar foods.
- Eat the protein on your plate first. You're less likely to eat starchy foods afterward, and your body burns more calories while digesting protein than fat or carbs—a concept called the "thermic effect of food."[138]

Another way to lose weight is through meal-replacement shakes. These provide a filling and nutritious beverage in place

---

[137] Habiba Samreen and Suneela Dhaneshwar, "Artificial Sweeteners: Perceptions and Realities," *Current Diabetes Reviews* 19, no. 7 (2023): 1–14, e290422204241, https://doi.org/10.2174/1573399818666220429083052.

[138] Manuel Calcagno et al., "The Thermic Effect of Food: A Review," *Journal of the American College of Nutrition* 38, no. 6 (2019): 547–551, https://doi.org/10.1080/07315724.2018.1552544.

of at least one meal of the day. Avoiding one meal decision spares you from making a bad choice or even the stress of having to decide. Strongly encouraged or mandatory group sessions often go along with this, providing the social benefit patients get from structured meal replacement programs.[139] Like with exercise, the social impact of group sessions during intense dietary changes helps individuals commiserate with others experiencing the same restrictions. Patients can share coping strategies and words of encouragement or simply listen to each other vent about how difficult it can be to maintain a normal life while getting nutrition from protein shakes.

At some point, however, you'll need to transition back to regular foods from meal-replacement shakes. This leads some to simply use a calorie-reduced diet from the beginning. Which is the magical diet that offers the best results? Naturally, it depends. Some individuals find they can control their appetite with a low-carb, high-fat-and-protein diet. This can reverse insulin resistance and diabetes by "freeing space" to store sugar while burning the liver fat contributing to insulin resistance. This is most effective with a calorie-reduced diet because it forces the body to look "inward" for stored energy to burn. Patients on insulin and certain diabetic medications should make dietary changes with medical guidance in order to avoid hypoglycemia.

A ketogenic diet ("keto") takes the low-carb and high-fat program to the extreme. This leads the body to burn fat and ketones for energy. The liver produces ketones when insulin levels are low and fat is available—people often report subjec-

---

[139] Jamy D. Ard et al., "Effectiveness of a Total Meal Replacement Program (OPTIFAST Program) on Weight Loss: Results from the OPTIWIN Study," *Obesity* 27, no. 1 (January 2019): 22–29, https://doi.org/10.1002/oby.22303.

tive benefits on mood and energy when this happens. A huge number of books and other resources exist on the ketogenic diet. To be brief, some find it extremely effective for controlling their appetite, reversing diabetes, and generally feeling well. Others are sensitive to changes in saturated fat, and keto requires an increase in the total amount of fat a person eats. This *may* increase the risk of heart disease by increasing the particles that carry LDL cholesterol ("bad cholesterol") in some people.[140] A potential workaround is prioritizing foods like avocados, olive oil, seeds, and nuts with lean meats for protein.

These modifications create a commonly recommended balanced diet, the Mediterranean diet:

- High intake of fruits and vegetables, which are rich in vitamins, minerals, antioxidants, and fiber.
- Olive oil is a primary source of fat in the Mediterranean diet and is rich in monounsaturated fatty acids and antioxidants.
- Fish and seafood consumed in moderation provide a good source of protein and omega-3 fatty acids.
- Legumes including beans, chickpeas, and lentils are good sources of protein and fiber.
- Nuts and seeds are a good source of healthy fats, protein, and fiber.
- Moderate consumption of dairy products, including cheese and yogurt, which provide calcium and protein.

The diet also recommends low or moderate intake of red meat but relatively high intake of whole grains like breads and pastas. Individuals following a low-carb diet may replace whole

---

[140] Damian Dyńka et al., "The Ketogenic Diet and Cardiovascular Diseases," *Nutrients* 15, no. 15 (2023): 3368, https://doi.org/10.3390/nu15153368.

grains with dietary fiber in nuts, seeds, fruits, and vegetables. After bariatric surgery, tough meats and nuts/seeds are some of the last foods to be reintroduced because they're more difficult to digest.

Weight Loss Medications

Anti-obesity medications (AOMs) are often an early first intervention for a medical weight loss program before bariatric surgery. Ideally, these are used with other lifestyle recommendations. AOMs are necessary tools in managing obesity and work through different pathways, typically within the hypothalamus in the brain, which controls appetite.

Many of the genes that predispose individuals to obesity code for proteins in the brain and hypothalamus, specifically, so these medications are an opportunity to level the playing field. Some physicians and patients may be reluctant to turn to medications for weight loss without first spending months or years dieting and exercising. However, this becomes a "two steps forward, three steps back" relationship for many because of the biological mechanisms that promote regaining weight. These medications—and resistance training—help prevent biology from undoing weight loss. Note: due to potential interactions with anesthesia and surgical risk, many surgeons/anesthesiologists may require weaning off AOMs shortly before surgery.

Testosterone Replacement

We discussed hormonal replacement therapies in Chapter 2, including the risks and benefits for different populations. Men with obesity often suffer from low free (active) testosterone, even after improving their lifestyle. This makes weight loss more difficult, slows recovery from exercise, and directly limits building muscle mass.[141]

Men with prostate disease/cancer, certain blood disorders, and untreated sleep apnea may not be good candidates for testosterone therapy. But others may use this treatment to help them lose weight, have more energy, and increase their physical activity. These changes can break the cycle of obesity causing low testosterone, and improving metabolic health may restore testosterone levels. However, prolonged testosterone supplementation may have the opposite effect and suppress the hormonal control pathways for testosterone production.

NEUROPSYCHIATRIC AND SLEEP

Candidates for bariatric surgery undergo an initial psychological evaluation to identify any risks that would increase the odds of a poor outcome from surgery. These include depression, anxiety, and addictive behaviors. Regarding depression and anxiety, these are risks for poor outcomes of most surgery types because they often come with inadequate nutrition, lower rates of exercise, poor sleep, and other downstream effects.

Despite the safety of these procedures, the bariatric surgery journey is profoundly life altering. A person must change many aspects of their life, including the way they eat, supplements they take, frequency of medical appointments they must attend, and their appearance. These expected stressors can provoke or worsen mood disorders. If a surgical complication forces another

---

141 Marie Sinclair et al., "Testosterone Therapy Increases Muscle Mass in Men with Cirrhosis and Low Testosterone: A Randomised Controlled Trial," *Journal of Hepatology* 65, no. 5 (November 2016): 906–913, https://doi.org/10.1016/j.jhep.2016.06.007; Atsumu Yuki et al., "Relationship Between Low Free Testosterone Levels and Loss of Muscle Mass," *Scientific Reports* 3 (2013): 1–5, 1818, https://doi.org/10.1038/srep01818.

hospital stay or a complete pause of food intake by mouth, the stress is only that much greater—though this specific risk is very low.[142]

Addiction and bariatric surgery have an interesting relationship. Likely due to changes in alcohol absorption and loss of eating as either a compensatory or reward behavior, patients after bariatric surgery have a higher risk of alcoholism. The prehab process involves screening for and educating about the risk of substance addiction after surgery.

Mood

Managing the risks of some conditions most commonly associated with obesity usually involves antidepressants like SSRIs, SNRIs, and atypical antidepressants. The combination medication bupropion/naltrexone (Qsymia) can address multiple problems at once. The naltrexone side may reduce addictive behaviors, while the bupropion improves mood symptoms.[143] Together, they also significantly support weight loss. Individuals will often complement these medical therapies with psychiatric therapy ("talk therapy") for added benefit. As introduced earlier, these SNRIs may help nerve pain from diabetic neuropathy or other causes as well.

---

142 A. Van Gossum et al., "Home Parenteral Nutrition (HPN) in Patients with Post-Bariatric Surgery Complications," *Clinical Nutrition* 36, no. 5 (October 2017): 1345–1348, https://doi.org/10.1016/j.clnu.2016.08.025.

143 Wissam Ghusn et al., "Weight-Centric Treatment of Depression and Chronic Pain," *Obesity Pillars* 3 (September 2022): 1–8, 100025, https://doi.org/10.1016/j.obpill.2022.100025.

Pain

Chronic pain and obesity have a bidirectional relationship. Pain often contributes to worsening obesity due to inactivity and problematic eating behaviors, and obesity increases inflammation and stress on painful joints.[144] In addition, obesity worsens diabetes, which is one of the main causes of painful neuropathy.

In bariatric surgery prehabilitation, pain management often addresses multiple issues and includes medication for improving mood and neuropathic pain. This can include a combination of remedies found in Chapter 2—most commonly gabapentinoids, NSAIDs, locally injected corticosteroids, platelet-rich plasma (PRP), or hyaluronic acid. Other less common (but situationally more effective) neuropathic pain meds like oxcarbazepine may impact weight less than gabapentinoids.[145] In certain cases, medications like ketamine, cannabis, or opioids are included.

Most surgeons require stopping medical cannabis prior to surgery due to potential risks. If the pain remains after surgery, patients are instructed to minimize NSAIDs and likely opioids. NSAIDs increase the risk of stomach bleeding and ulcers along the surgical site with long-term use (not short term postoperatively), and opioids may worsen nausea and slow intestinal function.

Exercise is a critical method for relieving pain, especially nonspecific pain without an obvious injury like chronic back pain. Exercise avoidance to keep pain from worsening is just another aspect of the vicious cycle of obesity and pain. Simply

---

144 Francis Berenbaum et al., "Osteoarthritis, Inflammation and Obesity," *Current Opinion in Rheumatology* 25, no. 1 (January 2013): 114–118, https://doi.org/10.1097/BOR.ob013e32835a9414.

145 P. Magenta et al., "Oxcarbazepine Is Effective and Safe in the Treatment of Neuropathic Pain: Pooled Analysis of Seven Clinical Studies," *Neurological Sciences* 26, no. 4 (October 2005): 218–226, https://doi.org/10.1007/s10072-005-0464-z.

exercising with trained guidance to ensure proper technique can significantly improve pain and fear-avoidant behaviors. Exercise is a core treatment for conditions like fibromyalgia that occur more commonly with obesity. Patients should expect short-term increases in pain; however, in the long term, exercise reduces the heightened pain sensation.

Sleep

Patients with obesity have a much higher risk of obstructive sleep apnea (OSA) that worsens with higher BMIs due to changes in the neck and upper airway. Some think of this as a condition of sleepiness and minor inconvenience, but the long-term effects can be extreme—high blood pressure, diabetes, heart attack, stroke, and sleepiness-related accidents. Most patients with obesity benefit from a screening test for OSA like the Berlin or STOP-BANG questionnaires. These can determine if suspicion for OSA is enough to need a full sleep-study, either in a sleep lab or at home.

Pain and depression can cause poor sleep directly. Treating these may improve sleep as a result. Similarly, exercise is a great way to relieve general pain, and it can also dramatically improve the quality of sleep and reduce the time to fall asleep. Benzodiazepine sedatives like clonazepam (Klonopin), triazolam (Halcion), temazepam (Restoril), and others may worsen sleep apnea. Opioid pain medications may have a similar effect. Medications like trazodone may improve sleep quality in patients with OSA.

EXPECTATION MANAGEMENT

Before surgery, patients try to find the best nutrition and exercise plans for weight loss. For many patients, exercise alone will not lead to long-term weight loss. While exercise is still the most important intervention for maximum health benefits and weight maintenance, nutrition must be optimized to initiate weight loss.

Patient expectations also must be realistic. The path from considering surgery all the way to postoperative success is long and requires major lifestyle changes, and the list of potential complications is extensive. Fortunately, serious complications are actually quite rare. Several hurdles along the way can delay or derail surgery, including poor access to bariatric specialists and insurance-mandated waiting periods that may stretch the time from initial consultation to surgery to over six months.

Those unfamiliar with the process may snidely regard bariatric surgery as "the easy way out." Part of preparation is knowing that isn't the case and learning to tune out the misinformed. Even with a months-long preparatory period, mandatory evaluations, and presurgical weight loss, success rates are not 100 percent.

Weight loss specialists stress the lifestyle changes patients *must* make and maintain well before surgery takes place. For example, after surgery, patients should avoid NSAIDs, minimize alcohol intake, and diligently prevent nutritional deficiencies through supplementation. Resistance training and high-protein diets are essential to maximize muscle and bone density during rapid weight loss. The changes ultimately become second nature, but this evolution takes effort and time.

PREOPERATIVE SCREENING

Extensive and ongoing screening tests are a part of bariatric surgery that interested individuals must accept. Here's an overview of some general elements.

- Complete blood count (CBC) and important nutrients for red blood cell production and neurologic health—B12, folic acid, and ferritin/TIBC. The CBC and "coagulation panel" are standard preoperative tests to assess risk of bleeding.
- Fat-soluble vitamins and minerals and related values— Vitamin D, calcium, parathyroid hormone, vitamin A, zinc, copper, selenium, and potentially vitamin E and thiamine (B1).
- Hemoglobin A1C to check diabetes or insulin resistance, along with cholesterol and kidney function tests.

DELAY SURGERY REQUIREMENT

As surgery in this case intends to meet the goal of obesity and metabolic disease remission, an individual can "delay surgery" by making progress to this goal nonsurgically. Newer AOMs like semaglutide and tirzepatide are supporting weight loss that, for some, rivals surgical outcomes. These medications can stave off obesity but don't yet represent a durable (permanent) cure.

COMMON AND POTENTIAL COMPLICATIONS

As with any surgery, complications are something to be anticipated before the surgery takes place. Because many types of bariatric surgery are quite major, the complications can affect a few different bodily systems.

Hyperemesis is severe nausea and vomiting after bariatric

surgery. Things like ulcers, bowel blockage, and narrowing of the stomach sleeve can cause this vomiting, which may dangerously stress the GI tract, the superficial incision on the skin, or the internal incision along the stomach/intestines related to the procedure.[146]

Marginal ulceration, or ulcers on the stomach or intestine along the incision, is another similar complication after surgery. Although they're relatively uncommon, these usually present with heartburn and vomiting as long as the ulcer hasn't torn (perforated). Smoking is the major risk factor most stressed by surgeons. Treatment is conservative if the ulcer isn't perforated or bleeding, but severe cases require surgery.

Kidney stones and gallstones are another possible complication due to changes in urine and the flow of bile, respectively. As we've mentioned, nutritional deficiency is another major complication, which in specific cases may cause neuropathy and encephalopathy (brain dysfunction). When these occur, they are often from B vitamin deficiencies, and supplements can halt progression once detected.

Appetite suppression and smaller stomach capacity after surgery by design leads to eating less. Not getting enough critical vitamins and minerals is an important complication to monitor. The complications stemming from not consuming enough of specific vitamins and minerals are many and potentially severe, even irreversible. So expect to be on a list of supplements for the rest of your life. Your surgeon will provide a detailed supplementation regimen designed to prevent deficiencies.

Weight regain is another complication that individuals

---

[146] Usha K. Coblijin et al., "Symptomatic Marginal Ulcer Disease After Roux-en-Y Gastric Bypass: Incidence, Risk Factors and Management," *Obesity Surgery* 25 (2015): 805–811, https://doi.org/10.1007/s11695-014-1482-9.

avoid by being proactive. This is necessary and usually involves continuing the same exercise regimen from prehab with an even greater focus on resistance training. More muscle mass maintains a higher metabolic rate, which keeps the body from reducing calorie needs and slowing weight loss. We want to promote this positive cycle as much as possible after surgery. The good news is that weight loss will likely improve exercise tolerance and pain levels.

It's important to intervene after surgery when weight loss stops and not wait until you *regain* weight to do something. We call this starting at the plateau, or when weight loss tapers off. This strategy will ultimately result in a lower final weight and should involve guidance from your weight loss specialist. At this time, your team may prescribe changes in nutrition, exercise, or weight loss medications. The minute you stop losing weight, seek additional guidance to keep from regaining weight. This does not mean you are doomed to yo-yo back to a prior weight— *that* level of hypervigilance and anxiety will not benefit you!

That final point paints the picture of bariatric surgery. No, it's not a quick and easy fix for people suffering from obesity and metabolic issues, but the journey before, during, and after bariatric surgery is not unmanageable either. Proper planning and dedication make bariatric surgery a great option for so many people to permanently change their lives and start their healthier, more active future.

This journey doesn't technically even have a finish line. Think of surgery as the transition to a new lifestyle. It makes keeping to a healthy diet and following good exercise principles easier to maintain. Let surgery be the facilitator that helps you lose weight and reach your goals.

ACTION POINTS

- Bariatric surgery is a long road and far from an easy fix. There are requirements and conditions before a patient will be appropriate for surgery. Due to how most bariatric procedures work, the way the body absorbs nutrients will be permanently changed afterward.
- The bariatric surgery treatment team is diverse and plays a role in every aspect of a patient's life. The team works together to make the patient a better candidate for surgery and reduce risks. Included in this is also making sure that patients will be in a place—physically, mentally, and emotionally—to continue losing weight after surgery.
- Exercise on its own, particularly steady aerobic exercise, is not the ideal strategy to lose weight before bariatric surgery. An ideal method is to combine aerobic and resistance exercise with a nutritional plan that stresses high protein intake and a calorie deficit. As with all prehab, the plan is only effective if it can be followed. A patient's prehab regimen must be unique and tailored to their needs, and there is more than one way to be successful.
- A patient's expectations before bariatric surgery should be realistic. The surgery is something that makes weight loss easier, but it doesn't perform the full scope of work for the patient. Although serious complications are rare, there are many potential complications that can arise and a new lifestyle that must be diligently followed.

CHAPTER 6

AMPUTEE PREHABILITATION

DECIDING TO PROCEED AHEAD WITH A NON-EMERGENT AMPU-tation is one of the most difficult decisions a person can be faced to make. Whether this is necessitated by blood vessel disease, an unhealing wound, or any other reason, it is natural to struggle immensely when coming to terms with a sudden change to one's body image and function. Nothing written here can take away from that psychological adjustment, and there is no quick fix—facing amputation is a transformative battle.

This doesn't mean all hope is lost or that amputation due to metabolic disease is simply inevitable. We have strategies available that will slowly but steadily improve a person's quality of life, and in some cases, these tactics *may* even prevent an amputation from needing to occur.[147]

There are case reports of fasting programs halting progression of chronic wounds and diabetic complications that could have led to amputations. It is possible for supervised intensive fasting programs to reverse diabetes. Many people aren't aware of the non-pharmacological methods for potentially reversing or slowing the most common conditions that lead to amputations.

The data for these types of remedies is often limited to case reports (basically, formal anecdotes) because funding and structuring clinical trials would be difficult. If the option were on the table, could you dig down deep to potentially save a toe, foot, or limb? And if that weren't possible, what measures would you take to receive the best prosthetic possible?

This chapter will detail what can be done to strive for the best possible outcomes, or even potentially avoid amputation. Not all amputations allow time for preparation. The prehabilitation processes that best prepare for or prevent an amputation and what comes next are key for making the most of this difficult situation.

TREATMENT TEAM AND HELPFUL TERMINOLOGY

The specialized team for amputation guides preparation, the procedure, and rehabilitation after surgery. The recovery after amputation is far more complicated than fitting a prosthetic and becoming comfortable wearing it. It takes many steps and months or years of physical therapy. For that reason, the treat-

---

147 Craig Boerner, "New Procedure Helps Patients Avoid Leg Amputations," *VUMC News*, March 30, 2023, https://news.vumc.org/2023/03/30/new-procedure-helps-patients-avoid-leg-amputation/; Robert G. Frykberg et al., "Surgical Strategies for Prevention of Amputation of the Diabetic Foot," *Journal of Clinical Orthopaedics and Trauma* 17 (June 2021): 99–105, https://doi.org/10.1016/j.jcot.2021.02.019; Mark A. Creager et al., "Reducing Nontraumatic Lower-Extremity Amputations by 20% by 2030: Time to Get to Our Feet: A Policy Statement From the American Heart Association," *Circulation* 143, no. 17 (2021): e875–e891, https://doi.org/10.1161/CIR.0000000000000967; Zoltan Kender et al., "Six-Month Periodic Fasting Does Not Affect Somatosensory Nerve Function in Type 2 Diabetes Patients," *Frontiers in Endocrinology* 14 (2023): 1–12, 1143799, https://doi.org/10.3389/fendo.2023.1143799; Benjamin D. Horne et al., "Relation of Routine, Periodic Fasting to Risk of Diabetes Mellitus, and Coronary Artery Disease in Patients Undergoing Coronary Angiography," *American Journal of Cardiology* 109, no. 11 (2012): 1558–1562, https://doi.org/10.1016/j.amjcard.2012.01.379.

ment team might feel back-loaded with specialists who help with recovery and empower amputees' return to fulfilling lives.

SURGICAL TEAM

The first players to mention are the surgical team. This varies by hospital, but they generally include vascular, orthopedic, and/or podiatric surgeons. Trauma surgeons may also be involved depending on the events leading to amputation, but not typically in cases with time for prehab.

PHYSICAL MEDICINE

A physiatrist (physical medicine & rehabilitation specialist) often leads the rehabilitation team. In this context, this physician cares for individuals who have undergone limb amputations, optimizing pain control and prescribing therapies designed to improve function and mobility status. Physiatrists are trained in assessing patients for assistive device (cane, walker, etc.) and prosthetic needs based on current and expected capabilities. They work closely with the prosthetics team to assess prosthetic fit and postsurgical limb health.

Finally, physiatrists often oversee pain management by personalizing a pain-control regimen with multiple approaches before and after surgery. This provides the best chance of getting back to independent physical functioning and the ability to participate in therapy services. Adequate pain control prior to amputation improves the likelihood of reduced or absent phantom limb pain.

OTHER MEDICAL MANAGEMENT

The medical management team is responsible for a patient's health status before surgery. For example, endocrinologists help tightly control patients' blood sugar to support wound healing and minimize complications. The vascular team evaluates the patients' artery disease and offers interventions to potentially delay amputation, optimize remaining limb length, and improve postoperative wound healing.

BEHAVIORAL HEALTH

Ideally, a psychologist should meet with a patient and their family to identify emotions and unspoken fears that come with undergoing an amputation. They assess the patient's social support, attend to caregiver concerns, emphasize healthy coping responses, and address any mood disorders that may worsen after limb loss.

NUTRITIONAL TEAM

Registered dieticians are important because diet, particularly sugar, may make a big difference when it comes to amputations. These professionals optimize nutrition before the procedure to maximize wound healing, especially protein intake and carbohydrate control in patients with diabetes.

PROSTHETICS AND ORTHOTICS (P&O) SPECIALIST

The certified prosthetist recommends the best prosthesis type for a patient's mobility needs after an amputation surgery. They identify orthotic solutions—bracing, inserts, etc.—that help prevent secondary conditions. This process involves structuring a timeline for early prosthetic fitting and training.

REHABILITATION THERAPISTS

As introduced earlier, physical and occupational therapists develop a customized treatment plan that maximizes functional independence before and after surgery. They train patients in using assistive devices, modifying environments, transferring between bed and wheelchair, and remaining limb care. They practice techniques with patients to help them adapt to daily living, including dressing, grooming, and managing the ins and outs of daily life. They design programs for maintaining mobility, activity, and range of motion in affected limbs. They also focus on preserving strength and function and anticipating any challenges that might show up after amputation surgery.

Vocational rehabilitation counselors aid patients in identifying work opportunities that match their individual skills, abilities, and interests. They also coordinate training opportunities and job placement resources and ensure workplace environment accessibility. Recreational therapists also help interested patients find opportunities for participating in adaptive sports. Some examples are sled hockey, skiing, surfing, billiards, rock climbing, bowling, wheelchair basketball, fishing, sailing, mountain biking, horseback riding, wheelchair rugby, dragon boat racing, curling, and golf.

CARE OVERVIEW

The sequence of steps through which patients undergoing amputation must transition starts with an initial discussion and continues all the way through surgery and an extensive postoperative recovery period.

Care will differ between elective and emergency amputations. In emergency situations, obviously there isn't time for most of the steps we referenced. For our purposes, let's focus on planned amputation surgeries with time for a prehabilitation period—though the postoperative periods will be similar in both scenarios. The most common causes of *planned* amputations are blood vessel diseases and nonhealing foot ulcers from risk factors like diabetes, smoking, infections, and congenital defects. Over 80 percent of all amputations in the United States are due to vascular causes, which may allow for this longer prehabilitation period. Ninety-seven percent of these cases involve lower extremities. Conditioning before and after surgery tends to be limited due to older age, comorbidities that prevent physical activity, and reduced motivation from depression.[148] Overcoming these obstacles is a huge part of better outcomes and quality of life after surgery.

Even for patients with gradually progressing blood vessel diseases, amputation surgery timing can still be unpredictable. Specialists have noted in patient focus groups that patients often delay seeking medical care until poor blood flow progresses to severe pain, ulcers, and tissue death. Most other prehab scenarios in this book recommend at least six weeks of preparation time using the prehab pillar components. This becomes very difficult to accomplish if patients don't present for medical care until they're unable to walk. Even if the surgery is planned months in advance, minor procedures could take place

---

[148] Edwin N. Aroke et al., "Perioperative Considerations for Patients with Major Depressive Disorder Undergoing Surgery," *Journal of PeriAnesthesia Nursing* 35, no. 2 (April 2020): 112–119, https://doi.org/10.1016/j.jopan.2019.08.011.

during the prehab period and disrupt exercise regimens. Despite these challenges, successful prehab programs can make a major difference before surgery.

Similar to any planned surgery, individuals undergoing limb amputation go through a screening process before prehab begins. Anemia and diet are important parts of this screening. A registered dietician optimizes caloric intake and protein consumption to promote wound healing and muscle mass. Cigarette smokers should quit at this time. Lab testing also checks a patient's risk for surgical complications from malnutrition, anemia, or uncontrolled diabetes.

A preoperative physical exam of all extremities occurs early. Sensation testing in the hands and feet may identify peripheral neuropathy. The physical exam also tests functional mobility, gait, and balance. This comes in handy later when prescribing assistive devices and fitting prosthetics. Existing wounds on all limbs need assessment, measuring size, color, and skin temperature. Joint integrity, strength, and range of motion are important details as well. Hand strength and fine motor skills inform whether a patient will be able to independently use a manual wheelchair or prosthesis.

Presurgical assessment also includes baseline evaluation of functional status, psychological profile, social barriers to care, and rehabilitation goals. The physical portions of this exam help design individualized treatment plans that align with abilities and goals after surgery. This helps anticipate the most likely complications, allowing the treatment team to use techniques to clear those obstacles or at least make them less likely.

This process often includes ways to make patients better candidates for surgery. If we help a person become healthier by lowering their blood sugar and addressing other comorbidities like damaged blood vessels, we lower the risk of bad surgical outcomes. All else held equal, the higher a patient's presurgical function is, the more advanced the prosthetic they will be qualified to receive. This isn't even just because insurance companies look for any reason to spend less money; an overly complicated prosthetic often just sits in the closet unused. With limited mobility, patients likely function *better* using a basic device than one with a fancy microchip knee, for example.

If your goal is the greatest mobility and most advanced prosthetic possible, take prehab seriously. How you prepare before surgery impacts everything that comes after.

PREHABILITATION PILLARS: AMPUTATION

Preoperative preparation for patients undergoing limb amputation procedures is a complex and under-researched area of prehabilitation. This is largely due to the circumstances that make amputations necessary and the comorbidities of populations likely to need this procedure. Limb amputations are life-changing events that require higher physical energy and psychological engagement to maximize independent functional movements. Because of this, the prehab period before surgery lays the foundation for strong recovery and better quality of life after surgery.

EXERCISE

Regular physical activity can increase aerobic capacity and muscle mass and reverse prediabetes and diabetes. On the other hand, poor fitness scores and inability to move freely before surgery worsens surgical risks and physical weakness after the procedure and extends the time before patients can participate in rehabilitation.

Patients undergoing amputations need exercise programs personalized to their physical capabilities. Comorbidities and functional limitations from pain, impaired balance, or existing limb deformity can make participation in standard exercise difficult. Research specifically for individuals before amputations is limited, but for other types of major surgery, exercise during prehab leads to fewer complications, shortened time in the hospital, and minimized postoperative functional decline. Again, this comes back to one of the root principles of prehab—put in the hard work upfront to make recovery quicker and easier.

Ideally, patients will engage in at least thirty minutes of moderate intensity exercise a day. If a patient is able, high-intensity interval training (HIIT) is a great method to boost aerobic exercise ability in a short window of time. Remember, exercise intensity level is *very* relative; high intensity for one person could be a literal walk in the park for another. Use this to your advantage...but under close supervision.

Closed chain, compound exercises like squats, deadlifts, or anything that works multiple muscle groups at once are more effective than exercises that only work individual muscles. This isn't realistic for all patients preparing for amputation. In such cases, open chain exercises that isolate one muscle group, like machine-based leg extensions or dumbbell bicep curls, can still be effective, especially if paired with exercises targeting the antagonist muscles. This would be like performing bicep curls followed by triceps press or leg curls and leg extensions. This increases blood flow into the limb and "balances" the muscles controlling a single joint.

Another modification for resistance training relies on isometric exercises where the muscle groups remain active but stationary in a working position. Exercises like planks and wall sits require less dynamic balance and are less prone to causing injury.[149] This is important because patients should exercise despite already having had prior amputations that could negatively affect balance. Isometric exercise may be safer and easier to perform in these situations.

Just like HIIT, other aerobic exercise is beneficial when possible, even if that means "just" walking. Aerobic training makes existing muscles and tissues more efficient at extracting oxygen from blood and producing energy. Many people facing amputation have impaired circulation. Aerobic exercise increases levels of certain hormones that tell the body to generate new blood vessels while also making muscles better at using the blood already reaching them.[150]

Again, aerobic exercise comes back to doing what you're able to do safely. Using the elliptical is much easier than the treadmill for some people. That's fine—it's still exercise. Aquatic therapy can be very beneficial because the warm water dilates the blood vessels and temporarily increases circulation. Supervision during exercise, especially in water, is key. Circulatory issues overall lead to a higher risk of muscle cramping, and open wounds may prevent water therapies. Also, medical clearance before starting an exercise routine is important. If a person has vascular disease in limbs, they likely also have some degree of heart disease. Only a proper medical exam—potentially with a stress test—can clear patients for exercise and make sure that

---

149 Biggie Baffour-Awuah et al., "An Evidence-Based Guide to the Efficacy and Safety of Isometric Resistance Training in Hypertension and Clinical Implications," *Clinical Hypertension* 29 (2023): 1–12, 9, https://doi.org/10.1186/s40885-022-00232-3; Christopher Kevin Wong et al., "Exercise Programs to Improve Gait Performance in People with Lower Limb Amputation," *Prosthetics and Orthotics International* 40, no. 1 (February 2016): 8–17, https://doi.org/10.1177/0309364614546926.

150 Daniel J. Green and Kurt J. Smith, "Effects of Exercise on Vascular Function, Structure, and Health in Humans," *Cold Spring Harbor Perspectives in Medicine* 8, no. 4 (2018): 1–15, a029819, https://doi.org/10.1101/cshperspect.a029819.

"bad" arteries aren't going to cause angina (chest pain from the heart working harder) or something worse.

The best overarching strategy for patients preparing for amputation, similar to other prehab regimens, is progressive overload. This means gradually increasing the intensity of work your body is doing. When poor blood flow is in the mix, participants quickly reach a point where they have limb pain and performance rapidly drops. Gradually push yourself until you near the "I can't go any further" limit. Then rest. The next time you exercise, push yourself a little bit further. That way, over time, you nudge your exercise ceiling higher, promoting better blood flow and stimulating the production of new blood vessels. This may mean walking "sets" of a single city block and then resting. Eventually, you'd tolerate two blocks. Then three. Then five.

In many cases, exercise is as much about improving metabolic diseases like diabetes as adding muscle mass or improving bone density. With diabetes, resistance (strength) training is important because added muscle mass equals more storage "space" for blood sugar. Aerobic exercise helps the body quickly burn off excess circulating blood sugar. These go hand in hand and can even play a role in reversing prediabetes and diabetes. Of course, other lifestyle changes turbocharge this strategy's effectiveness.

LIFESTYLE

For most people, the most important early change to make is switching to a high protein, low carbohydrate diet. A supervised fasting program may also be beneficial for many. Any potential extra "strain" on the kidneys from high-protein diets (a relationship still open to debate) is likely less of a concern. High protein supports muscle, and these calories often replace refined carbohydrates in the diet—irrefutably a win during prehabilitation.

Nutrition provides key energy needed for prehab and rehabilitation therapy, promotes muscle repair, and supports postoperative wound healing. It also plays a role in slowing or even reversing the metabolic conditions that lead to many amputations. Individuals who are malnourished face worse surgical outcomes and postoperative quality of life because they lack the protein and access to stored energy necessary to cope with the stress of surgery.[151] A proper diet, as discussed above, makes exercise recovery more effective.

Early in prehab, a registered dietician should make sure a patient eats enough protein. They can also help work around special dietary needs—carb control for individuals with diabetes and even shopping and recipe guidance for convenience. For patients undergoing amputation, there aren't specific guidelines beyond these basics, but proper nutritional support can speed up recovery and physical activity benefits before and after surgery.

Cutting sugar from the diet isn't just important for controlling diabetes and blood vessel damage. This takes away a main "food" source for bacteria, so preoperative and postoperative infections may be less severe or avoided.

Quitting smoking is vitally important. Smoke is very inflammatory, damaging blood vessels. Nicotine is a vasoconstrictor, meaning it "tightens" the blood vessels and increases blood pressure. If someone has blood vessel disease, that means their blood vessels are already narrower than normal. Consuming nicotine is

---

[151] Aniek M. Kolen et al., "A Scoping Review on Nutritional Intake and Nutritional Status in People with a Major Dysvascular Lower Limb Amputation," *Disability and Rehabilitation* 46, no. 2 (2024): 257–269, https://doi.org/10.1080/09638288.2022.2164363.

just going to further narrow blood vessels and impair circulation. Quitting smoking is considered a requirement before surgery for amputation procedures more than just about anything else.

NEUROPSYCHIATRIC

Limb amputation is a life-changing event that can result in reduced mobility and independence. Psychological conditions or depression may appear or worsen after surgery. Interventions that deal with mood disorders are often just as important as exercise and lifestyle interventions. Dealing with such a dramatic and unwanted change to one's physical identity is difficult, and the medical team takes this pillar of prehab very seriously.

Pain control plays a major role in this pillar because a failure to control pain before surgery and immediately after may make chronic pain or phantom pain after surgery more likely.[152] Pain may not get to zero, but using medications and exercise to improve control is a top priority.

Adequate, quality sleep is always important during prehab, but in this case, sleep's main benefits are better blood sugar and blood pressure control. Poor sleep elevates stress hormones like cortisol and adrenaline, which worsen blood sugar. Quality sleep doesn't resolve issues overnight, but it helps gradually control the root causes.

Depression and "adjustment disorders" are quite common after amputation surgery. Amputation is a huge change, and one of the best ways to adapt is through therapy and peer support groups. Some amputations are more common than others. For example, vascular disease is much more likely to lead to

---

152 M. J. E. Neil, "Pain After Amputation," *BJA Education* 16, no. 3 (March 2016): 107–112, https://doi.org/10.1093/bjaed/mkv028.

amputation of lower extremities. Knowing that there are others going through this exact process and coping effectively can be quite helpful. Undergoing an amputation is likely to trigger many emotions, including anger, grief, and depression. Limb loss survivors are given space to recognize and identify these emotions. Heroic cheerfulness, or "suck it up stoicism," might be challenged under these circumstances as part of therapy because it likely masks the true emotions a survivor is feeling.

Therapy sessions are an important time to talk through unspoken fears a patient might have about the procedure and life after amputation. Sessions are a safe space for patients to speak about their fear of death, body image, social rejection, loss of independence, employment and housing issues, and changes in sexual function. Hearing caregiver concerns is important; what assistance the patient might need, how the procedure will impact their living situation or ability to provide income, and determining a care schedule are only some common concerns. This is a great time to introduce relaxation techniques, breathing exercises, meditation, mindfulness, and cognitive behavior therapies.

DELAY SURGERY REQUIREMENT

Imagine a freight train barreling down at you. What are the best ways to extend the railroad tracks so you have more time before it arrives? This vivid metaphor is similar to how many regard amputation surgery. What can be done to push that surgery as far into the future as possible?

As hinted at earlier, when an amputation procedure is planned far in advance, small things may help put off that major surgery. Sometimes these are artery bypasses or smaller amputations. For example, most people would prefer to lose a toe rather than an entire foot. Antibiotics and tighter diabetes control can support healing wounds and remove that sugars that bacteria love to eat. A progressive walking or exercise program is essential for improving mobility before surgery. Exercise and mobility have a whole host of benefits that can start a "virtuous cycle" toward making a person healthier and pushing amputation further into the future.

Finally, arguably the most aggressive nutritional treatment that may delay surgery involves fasting. Some outspoken clinicians have reported success with slowing and even reversing diabetes using low carbohydrate diets and extreme fasting programs combined with exercise.[153] This is not an easy or guaranteed solution, but knowing that metabolic conditions that lead to amputation can be slowed or even reversed is a great provider of hope. As of this writing, no large-scale studies have corroborated these reports; however, accumulating data connects fasting and diabetes resolution.[154] As improved blood sugar control benefits wounds, by extension, fasting may plausibly have this effect. Patients may potentially include fasting in their prehab plan with close guidance from medical professionals.

AMPUTATION AND PROSTHETIC TYPES

A full description of available technologies is extensive and subject to frequent revision; however, for completeness, it's worth

---

[153] Renza Scibilia, "The Diabetes Code: Prevent and Reverse Type 2 Diabetes Naturally," *Clinical Diabetes* 37, no. 3 (2019): 302–303, https://doi.org/10.2337/cd19-0025.

[154] Hongbo Zhang et al., "Alternate-Day Fasting Alleviates Diabetes-Induced Glycolipid Metabolism Disorders: Roles of FGF21 and Bile Acids," *Journal of Nutritional Biochemistry* 83 (September 2020): 108403, https://doi.org/10.1016/j.jnutbio.2020.108403; Sarah J. Hallberg et al., "Reversing Type 2 Diabetes: A Narrative Review of the Evidence," *Nutrients* 11, no. 4 (2019): 766, https://doi.org/10.3390/nu11040766.

discussing the basic major *nontraumatic* amputations and their corresponding prosthetic components.

Upper Extremity (Arm)

1. Transradial Amputation (Below Elbow)
   A. Prosthesis: Myoelectric prosthesis or body-powered prosthesis, which allows for hand and wrist movements. Myoelectric prosthesis uses sensors to pick up signals from the remaining nerves to tell the prosthetic when to move. These are often heavier than the body-powered prostheses and are more expensive to purchase and repair, but they can be impressively high-tech.
2. Transhumeral Amputation (Above Elbow)
   A. Prosthesis: Myoelectric prosthesis or body-powered prosthesis with elbow and hand functionality.

Lower Extremity

1. Transtibial Amputation (Below Knee)
   A. Prosthesis: Prosthetic limb with a socket, pylon (shaft), and foot, often with energy-storing (spring-like) feet to aid in walking.
2. Transfemoral Amputation (Above Knee)
   A. Prosthesis: Prosthetic limb with a socket, knee joint, pylon, and foot, designed to mimic natural knee and leg movements. Knee joints have different features to help simulate healthy knee mechanics.

These prostheses are designed to help restore function and improve quality of life by allowing as much independence and mobility as possible.

COMMON AND POTENTIAL COMPLICATIONS

Incidences of vascular diseases and diabetes increase with age. As such, the number of amputation surgeries for the geriatric population in the United States is predicted to increase as the general population ages. Individuals over sixty years old are already the most common patients undergoing lower limb amputation. Studies suggest that as age increases, the risk of complications and bad outcomes after surgery increases.

Two of the most common surgical complications are blood clots like deep vein thromboses or DVTs and infection. Phantom pain and surgical pain can also arise after surgery. Phantom pain or sensation is any pain or feeling that comes from a body part that is no longer there. Getting a handle on chronic pain during the prehab period is the best way to limit this after surgery.

It may seem obvious, but improper skin care after surgery can also lead to complications. Ingrown hairs and inadequately cleaning the area can cause infections, which we want to avoid at all times. Nonhealing wounds are also something to monitor. Failing to deal with or treat a nonhealing wound can, in the worst cases, lead to another surgery or losing more of a limb.

This ties to other negative outcome possibilities when you first receive your prosthetic. Fit is very important. This perfect fit may be elusive because the area can swell after surgery. Heart or kidney failure also contribute to swelling. Avoiding pressure points is key, and if an area at the top of the prosthetic is really tight and a lower area is loose, that pressure differential can lead to other skin problems. A "total contact" fitting prosthetic and frequently adjusting the layers of stockings underneath helps prevent irregular pressure points on limbs even in the setting of swelling.

Finally, contracture is a permanent tightening of muscles, tendons, and other tissue that shortens and stiffens joints. Positioning after surgery is really important. For example, putting a pillow under certain areas or leaving the knee or hip bent for too long can risk developing contracture. Without putting weight on the limb, it becomes difficult to reverse this, and you're left with a joint that doesn't fully extend. Hamstrings and hip flexors are particularly prone to contracture, so be mindful of how you position yourself.

WHAT TO EXPECT DURING RECOVERY

The rehab team plays a major role in the recovery process. After a surgeon performs the amputation, a rehab doctor (physiatrist) looks after a patient's immediate medical needs, including helping with pain and rehab planning. This immediate period is called pre-prosthetic training, using exercises to strengthen the entire body and practice transferring between wheelchair, beds, and other surfaces.

The first follow-up visit with a rehab doctor should ideally come within two weeks of leaving the hospital. This professional will help you determine when it's appropriate to take measurements and start prosthesis design, all while monitoring limb health. When you're ready, your rehab doctor (if available) will write the prosthesis prescription. In areas with limited medical access, a primary care doctor may order this with guidance from a prosthetist. Again, the type of prosthesis depends in large part on your mobility capabilities and how active you were before surgery.

The next step after the prosthesis is ordered is limb shaping and positioning. There will likely be swelling after surgery that can last weeks. Wrapping the limb will help decrease swelling and shape the residual limb. Your physical therapist will teach you how to wrap your limb. Once cleared by your surgeon, begin wrapping your remaining limb daily.

This also typically requires surgeon clearance, but the next step is to wear a "shrinker" sock or, less commonly, a removable plastic dressing to decrease swelling and help protect the remaining limb. Your physical therapist will teach positions and stretches designed to maintain flexibility. Shaping and positioning the limb is important because it helps prepare you for your prosthesis.

Part of recovery involves managing amputation-related pain. Pain or changing sensations can occur in the remaining part *or* absent part of the limb. Phantom limb sensations often arise in the form of itching, tingling, and cramping. Phantom limb pain can feel like burning, stabbing, electric shocks, or other sensations. Better control of presurgery pain in the affected limb typically results in less pain after surgery.[155]

While amputation-related pain is an unfortunate part of the process, there are a few methods to help regulate it. Pretreating with gabapentinoids, ketamine, serotonin and norepinephrine reuptake inhibitors (SNRIs), or the other nerve pain medications before surgery may prevent phantom pain after. Relaxation techniques, massaging the affected area, and nerve blocks are other treatment options. Desensitization techniques like tapping directly on the remaining sensitive area or mirror therapy can help with pain and prosthesis tolerance. Keep a journal of when you feel pain and how bad it is on each occasion. Phantom pain is common, but it is also manageable.

Skin care is another important piece of recovery. Inspect your skin daily, using a mirror to look at the bottom and back of your affected leg or arm. Individual cases may vary so it's important to be in close contact with your surgeon. However, anything involving pain, swelling, warmth, redness, drainage, fever, or chills could be a sign of infection. Once cleared by your surgeon,

---

[155] Neil, "Pain After Amputation," 107–112.

wash your limb nightly with mild soap and lukewarm water. Rinse the area without soaking, and then pat dry with a towel. Avoid rubbing the area, and don't shave or use lotions, creams, or moisturizers on the area unless your doctor tells you to.

Fitting and getting used to a prosthesis involves some trial and error. The rehab team will work with you to make changes or adjust your prosthesis during rehab. If outpatient, stay in communication with your rehab doctor and prosthetist during the recovery process so they can help with pain, skin issues, or prosthetic issues.

Lower limb amputation therapy follows a standard progression. Some of the priorities are moving from sitting to standing and getting comfortable with a wheelchair, walker, or crutches. After you receive the prosthesis, therapies move to learning how to put it on and take it off (*donning* and *doffing*), walking, and climbing stairs. For upper limb amputation, the first priority is regaining the ability to perform activities of daily living (ADLs) like dressing and bathing.

For multiple reasons, you are at increased risk of falling after an amputation. New medicines and changes in circulation might make you feel dizzy and lead to falls. When getting out of bed, sit for a few seconds before standing. If you have severe or constant symptoms of dizziness, call your doctor right away for evaluation and medication management.

The psychological impact of going through amputation and everything that follows can (but doesn't have to) be substantial. Amputation is a life-changing experience. One of the best remedies to fight any source of distress is a support group to lean on every step of the way. Sharing and forming an emotional bond with others with similar experiences is invaluable. Your rehab team and different organizations are there to help you at each point of this journey.

Here are a few helpful websites with resources and information about support groups.

www.amputee-coalition.org

www.nationalamputation.org

www.americanamputee.org

Amputation surgery is a major change or turning point in a patient's life, but that doesn't mean there is no reason for hope. In fact, the prospects of receiving the best prosthetic possible and returning to normal life are often two powerful motivators. Powering through recovery and getting back to what you love to do are the best ways to improve quality of life after an amputation. With a well-fitting prosthetic, good therapy, and lifestyle changes, you can have a very full and active life after limb loss.

ACTION POINTS

- Quitting smoking is extremely important for delaying the need for amputation or deferring it altogether. If you need help quitting, talk to your doctor. Minimize even secondhand smoke prior to surgery.
- Pay attention to your diet. Eat protein-rich foods throughout the day. Adding a protein supplement drink can be helpful, but the goal is to aim for roughly two grams of protein per kilogram of body weight daily (or approximately one gram per pound). Work with your doctor to improve blood sugar and blood pressure before surgery.
- Exercise daily. If possible, walk for thirty minutes each day. Work with a physical therapist to strengthen muscles using free weights, resistance bands, and machines. Attend occupational therapy sessions to learn how to use assistive devices and to modify workouts. Prioritize pain control to make participating in preoperative aerobic activity easier.

- Establish care with a prosthetist to learn about prosthetic options that match your desired level of activity. Schedule a time for postop prosthesis and/or assistive device fitting and training.
- Prepare mentally. Anticipate practical challenges that might arise after surgery. Name the emotions you feel about the procedure. List the activities you enjoy and your defining personality traits. Identify sources of strength during your recovery, and connect with others if you feel comfortable doing so.

CHAPTER 7

TRANSPLANT PREHABILITATION

SOME MAY BELIEVE FINDING AN ORGAN FOR TRANSPLANT IS AS "simple" as matching blood types and reserving an operating room. Instead, transplants require a thorough and complex matching process completed well before the procedure. If you're at all familiar with this process, you might wonder why doctors test your blood for obscure viruses you've likely never heard of. What do the viruses that cause mononucleosis ("mono") have to do with qualifying for a new organ? The truth is that seemingly minor things may make a huge difference in medications to take and whose organs you can receive.

Such factors don't always make it impossible to receive an organ. For example, say you're a perfect match for an organ, but you, like many, have a dormant cytomegalovirus (CMV) infection. There's a good chance you'll still receive the organ, but it could require certain medications after transplant.

Matching patients with organs is a complicated process because organs are precious resources. The overall supply is limited, and lists of patients seeking a transplant can be long. Unfortunately, not everyone will receive the organ they need. The number-one thing you can do is make yourself as good a candidate for transplantation as possible.

HOW IMPORTANT *IS* PREHABILITATION PRIOR TO TRANSPLANT?

Not everyone has time for prehab, as some individuals suffer catastrophic injury or illness that immediately launches them from good health to organ failure, urgently needing transplant. Alternatively, others may be burdened by a gradually weakening organ for years. Who will fare better with transplant? Often the first individual, as they went from baseline good health to the transplant table before experiencing significant effects in the body.

Obviously this is not the case for everyone, but take these two real examples. Mr. X was a previously healthy male who caught a rare viral infection that caused cardiomyopathy, or sick heart muscle. Mr. Y was around ten years younger and had a rare gene mutation that caused a toxic protein to build up in the liver. Mr. X was up and walking in rehab within a week or two of transplant. Mr. Y spent over four hundred days in the hospital, and after several weeks in rehab, he had to return back to the ICU due to multiple complications.

This is not to scare you into action or use someone's misfortune for entertainment value. Simply put, anything you can do to improve your candidacy may both help you qualify for an organ transplant and improve your quality of life leading up to surgery. Frankly, transplant prehab is an endurance game. This chapter details preparation, treatment, and recovery for transplant candidates, with emphasis on specific prehabilitation measures that may truly impact how soon you qualify for transplantation and how rich your life will be afterward.

TREATMENT TEAM AND HELPFUL TERMINOLOGY

The "big four" solid organ transplants are kidney, liver, heart, and lung. Pancreas transplants are rarer, and sometimes other organs are transplanted.

Again, organs are presently a limited resource, meaning that simply getting approved for a new organ involves clearance from a panel of specialists. Everyone on the panel essentially weighs in on the patient's likelihood of success with the transplant procedure and recovery based on their health status and how well they've adhered to health and lifestyle recommendations along the way.

Depending on the organ in question, expect to interact with many of the following specialists.

SURGICAL AND MEDICAL SPECIALISTS

Transplant surgeons are often a subspecialist of a cardiothoracic surgeon (a specialist who performs surgery on organs inside the chest cavity—heart, lungs, etc.) or a general surgeon with fellowship training in liver, kidney, or other abdominal organ transplantation. Related to these team members, analogous medical counterparts like cardiologists, pulmonologists, and nephrologists focus on the heart, lungs, and kidneys. They often assume roles of presurgical medical management and long-term postoperative care of affected organ systems, with the surgical specialists more acutely involved during the period immediately before and after surgery. Endocrinologists, neurologists, hematologists, and other specialists may be involved as well, based on other medical conditions and complications.

NUTRITIONAL TEAM

Transplant nutritionists and registered dieticians are experts in nutrition and diagnosing malnutrition who anticipate typical nutritional complications that are unique to the transplant recipients. These professionals optimize nutrition to maximize wound healing, especially protein intake and carbohydrate control in patients with diabetes or malnutrition. They also help guide tube feeding recommendations for patients requiring supplemental nutrition.

REHABILITATION THERAPISTS

As introduced earlier, physical and occupational therapists develop a customized treatment plan that maximizes functional independence before and after surgery. They train patients in using assistive devices, modifying environments, transferring between bed and wheelchair, and performing remaining limb care. They practice techniques with patients to help them adapt to daily living, dressing, grooming, and managing the ins and outs of daily life. They design programs for maintaining mobility, activity, and range of motion in affected limbs. They also focus on preserving strength and function and anticipating any challenges that might show up after transplantation surgery.

- Respiratory therapist: A specialist who treats problems with lungs and breathing
- Psychologist/psychiatrist/neuropsychologist: Specialists in cognitive processes and behavior

- Palliative care team: A group of people who oversee relief and support for individuals with serious illnesses

Once a patient qualifies for an organ, how long does the waiting period last? Average wait times differ depending on the organ and region, but they usually fall in the ballpark of months to years, unfortunately.[156] This means the prehab period will almost certainly be longer for transplant surgery than for elective conditions like a knee replacement.

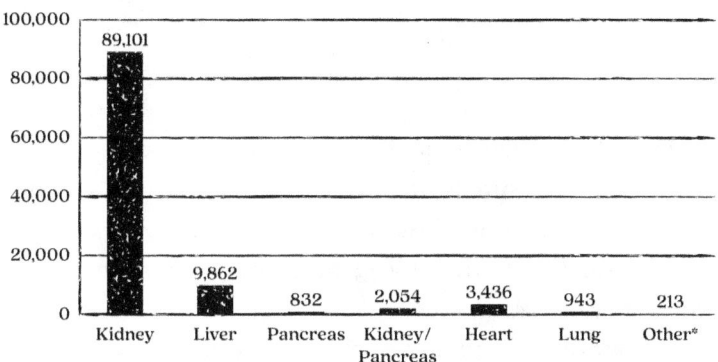

Patients on the Waiting List by Organ
As of March 2024

*Other includes kidney/pancreas and allograft transplants like face, hands, and abdominal wall.

Number of patients on the wait list for organ transplantation as of March 2024. Data provided by Organ Procurement and Transplantation Network (OPTN)

---

156 Darren Stewart et al., "Does Anybody Really Know What (the Kidney Median Waiting) Time Is?," *American Journal of Transplantation* 23, no. 2 (February 2023): 223–231, https://doi.org/10.1016/j.ajt.2022.12.005; Syed Shahyan Bakhtiyar et al., "Survival on the Heart Transplant Waiting List," JAMA *Cardiology* 5, no. 11 (2020): 1227–1235, https://doi.org/10.1001/jamacardio.2020.2795; Leonard E. Riley and Jorge Lascano, "Gender and Racial Disparities in Lung Transplantation in the United States," *Journal of Heart and Lung Transplantation* 40, no. 9 (September 2021): 963–969, https://doi.org/10.1016/j.healun.2021.06.004.

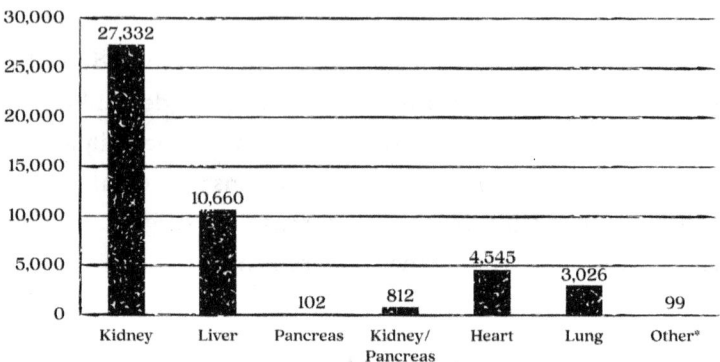

Transplants Performed by Organ
As of March 2024

*Other includes kidney/pancreas and allograft transplants like face, hands, and abdominal wall.

Based on OPTN data as of March 21, 2024. "Organ Donation Statistics," U.S. Health Resources & Services Administration, last reviewed March 2024, https://www.organdonor.gov/learn/organ-donation-statistics.

This may change in the future, should advances in bioengineering increase supply of organs or new medications reduce demand for organs. For instance, new medications like SGLT2 inhibitors and GLP-1 receptor agonists slow progression of heart and kidney disease.

Below are common causes of each type of organ failure.

- Heart: Congenital (from birth) issues, heart attacks, viral infections
- Lung: Smoking, work-related exposures (coal mining, for example), genetic conditions like cystic fibrosis or alpha-1 antitrypsin disease, autoimmune conditions like sarcoidosis, pulmonary fibrosis, pulmonary artery hypertension
- Liver: Metabolic dysfunction-associated steatotic liver disease (MASLD), viral infections, alcohol use, genetic conditions

- Kidney: High blood pressure, diabetes, genetic conditions like polycystic kidney disease, autoimmune conditions like lupus

CARE OVERVIEW

We've already established that transplant matching and procedures are complex processes. What follows is an overview of what to expect along the way.

The first step is screening and identifying the organ that is progressing toward organ failure. Spotting organ dysfunction or failure usually involves a primary care physician and medical specialists for that particular organ. For example, individuals with heart or kidney failure have likely been working with a cardiologist or nephrologist for years prior to needing transplantation. They will prescribe temporizing measures described later in the Delay Surgery Requirement section.

Next comes prehabilitation—making best use of lifestyle and medical interventions that include exercise, nutrition, proper medication use, and psychological conditions. A physiatrist, along with the treatment team, presents individualized prehab guidelines depending on the amount of time available before surgery and the patient's current health situation. For some chronic diseases, exercise will be limited by physical tolerance or due to medical risk.

Prehabilitation to improve a patient's readiness for transplant has become an essential phase of care for patients with end-stage organ disease. Frailty is a common comorbidity in this population and consists of deconditioning (inactivity), sarcopenia, and nutritional deficiencies.

Immediately following surgery, patients enter postoperative care and are managed by the transplant team who adjust antirejection medication dosages, monitor the new organ's function, and prevent infection. Transplantation-related issues and restrictions vary at this stage. For example, sometimes restrictions on weight bearing in the upper body are needed after chest surgery. After a patient clears surgery and immediate recovery, they transition to post-transplantation rehab either in an inpatient or outpatient setting. This involves changing their long-term lifestyle and learning how to manage their complex new medication regimen.

PREHABILITATION PILLARS: TRANSPLANTATION

Different organs come with different activity levels and types of safe exercise. Prehab for a kidney transplant is likely not the same as prehab for a heart or lung transplant. Prehab's goal—and main challenge—is to target risk factors for poor outcomes, as well as address the issues that lead to poor quality of life while a patient attempts to qualify for surgery.

This is no easy feat because failing organs affect the entire body's function. Just as bodily systems work together and depend on one another, so must the prehabilitation pillars—exercise, lifestyle, and neuropsychiatric.

EXERCISE

Exercise is absolutely encouraged during transplant prehabilitation but needs to be handled especially delicately. For instance, if patients are dealing with lung or heart failure, they are limited in the type of strength training they can do with their arms because resistance training may increase the back pressure on the heart. With a condition like chronic lung disease, where oxygen levels are lower than normal, aerobic exercise can drop those levels even lower. The body's response is to tighten the pulmonary arteries, which increases the blood pressure in those arteries—if excessive, this pulmonary hypertension can lead to heart failure as well.

This example isn't designed to scare you but to make you aware of the need to always monitor oxygen levels in the setting of chronic lung disease while exercising and to avoid doing anything to add further stress. This example also serves to illustrate the delicate balance in treatment plans your teams design. For these patients, when engaging in upper-body resistance training, limit the weight to five or ten pounds, and keep a constant eye on your oxygen with a pulse-ox finger monitor. Movements like crouching in a squatting position for too long can also raise pulmonary artery pressure. Participation in dedicated cardiac or pulmonary rehab will teach the unique consideration for each individual's personal condition.

For patients with kidney failure, exercise tolerance may be affected by electrolyte issues. These patients are more prone to things like high potassium or low sodium or magnesium. This can cause muscle cramping, nausea, and general discomfort, not to mention trouble maintaining healthy blood acid levels.

Exercise leads to the production of carbon dioxide, raising blood acidity. The kidneys and lungs primarily manage the blood's acidity, meaning that kidney or lung damage worsens exercise tolerance. They have less capacity to filter out waste, manage blood pH, and keep electrolytes balanced.

Exercise benefits the body by making muscles more efficient at pulling oxygen from the blood. It's not that the heart gets better at pumping or lungs get better at bringing in oxygen; primarily, the body gets better at using what it already has. That's why any exercise is beneficial during prehab. The main goal remains anticipating issues and personalizing exercise plans based on which organ is failing while not making matters worse or affecting other organs in the process.

In most cases, end-stage organ disease leads to low muscle mass (sarcopenia) and often low bone density too. Aerobic capacity is decreased as well, even when the lungs aren't the problem. Relative to prehab for other procedures, progress can be slow. Preventing even minor injuries is important so that progress isn't completely derailed. Blood-flow restriction training can be useful in these situations both to avoid using heavy weight and putting pressure on the heart and to reduce the chance of setting off chronic issues. However, the safety of this is highly person-dependent regarding the risk tolerance of the patient and treatment team. It's also important to note that steroids are often used in the short or intermediate term after a transplant. This risks provoking issues during rehab, particularly with muscle mass and blood sugar control.

Each condition also impacts muscle mass in different ways. Protein imbalance and wasting is common in kidney and liver disease. Chronic lung disease creates a "hypermetabolic state" that burns muscle. Heart failure's circulatory issues limit the exercise tolerance necessary for muscle maintenance.

If this sounds like a lot to wrap your head around, there's some good news. Cardiac and pulmonary rehab are outpatient physical therapy programs that focus on exercises that are safe for diseased hearts, lungs, and related systems. They are very good at monitoring oxygen levels and other diagnostics that can prevent issues that come with exercise. Sometimes, they even use EKG testing during sessions as an impromptu stress test, if needed. So you don't have to do this alone—programs like cardiac rehab are designed specifically for many of the purposes we've covered.

LIFESTYLE

Just like exercise, a patient's lifestyle recommendations are individualized to lead to the best possible outcomes. Often, these are tailored based on the organ in failure. For example, when kidney failure occurs, creatine monohydrate supplementation can be very beneficial for general quality of life—*especially* for individuals on dialysis—and can prevent cramping during exercise. Please review Chapter 2 for a more detailed discussion of benefits and misconceptions of creatine supplementation.

Other specific supplement recommendations are determined by deficiencies identified on lab testing. There is little broad advice other than making sure you take in enough macronutrients like protein, vitamins, and minerals to optimize health. Self-regulatory systems in the body may not work effectively when a person has organ failure, so your treatment team monitors vitamin and mineral levels with tests chosen specifically based on knowledge of common abnormalities in specific disease states. Vitamin D tends to be chronically low in patients with kidney disease; potassium and magnesium are often low for patients on certain heart medications. Medical professionals know this and prescribe supplements as needed to correct low values.

Like we've touched on throughout this book, quitting smoking is a major lifestyle adjustment that needs to happen before transplant surgery. Smoking contributes heavily to cardiovascular diseases, which are the most common cause of death for patients on dialysis. Despite this, smoking is still common among patients with kidney failure. Quitting smoking is an excellent step to get healthier, lower the risk of complications, and qualify for an organ. Many transplant programs won't even list a patient on a transplant waitlist if they continue to smoke, drink alcohol, or even refuse certain vaccines; as organs are considered a gift, certain sacrifices by recipients are necessary to ensure they are committed to caring for their new organ in the eyes of the team.

Nutritionally, tenets are similar as in other prehab scenarios. Unless specifically advised against, high-protein diets are crucial in the uphill battle for muscle maintenance. Carbohydrate restriction may help control metabolic disease, but for individuals with frailty, often the goal is to keep up with metabolic demand despite a poor appetite. If restricting carbohydrates makes foods unpalatable, any such restrictions would likely be relaxed.

NEUROPSYCHIATRIC

Some common conditions that cause a patient's organ failure often also cause neuropathy. Neuropathy (nerve dysfunction) is often a big issue within these medical populations. The main causes for liver failure are fatty liver disease and, less common these days, the hepatitis viruses. Fatty liver disease goes hand in hand with diabetes and neuropathy.

Kidney disease that leads to kidney failure is no exception, given the main causes of high blood pressure and diabetes. If diabetes is bad enough to cause kidney damage, it's usually bad enough to cause neuropathy. Neuropathic pain in the fingers and toes can present with burning, tingling, and diminished or absent sensation. Managing neuropathy is an important part of this pillar and makes a noticeable difference in quality of life during prehab. Some antirejection medications after transplant, such as tacrolimus, may cause neuropathy as well.

Depression is another important factor warranting attention. Conveniently, many of the medications that ease neuropathic pain are antidepressants. This makes it possible to treat the two conditions with one medication—always a plus. Similarly, patients awaiting transplant procedures often have sleep issues for reasons including decreased daytime activity making them less tired at night. Mood issues, pain, and stress also impair restful sleep, yet quality sleep is critical for resilience and recovery. Part of this process is screening for conditions like sleep apnea and promptly treating them. Unfortunately, some conditions and treatments related to organ failure, including orthopnea (shortness of breath when lying flat), CPAP/BiPAP machines, and overnight dialysis, may also impact sleep.

For those with mood issues and pain, addressing these often leads to better sleep. Lack of sleep will only worsen everything else—blood pressure and blood sugar, mood disorders, and most things that led to organ failure in the first place. However, dwelling on sleep difficulties can promote sleep anxiety and insomnia itself, so sleep medical or psychology specialists are often helpful.

Finally, the anticipatory anxiety leading up to transplant procedures can be intense on its own. Even with how far the science has come, these are still major surgeries with potential risks and complications. Depending on the organ and reason for transplant, recovery may be slow and prolonged, since waiting for transplant gradually depletes the body's resilience unless deliberately targeted. However, prehabilitation is a window of time to reclaim control of your health as much as possible. Regardless of the situation, you can turn things around and improve one step at a time. Change may be slow, but with steady diligence, it gets easier and eventually promotes substantial benefits.

EXPECTATION MANAGEMENT

Life after transplant may be radically different from life before the procedure. Early goal setting with step-by-step plans is a good way to prevent spontaneous "heroic" interventions with little benefit yet increased risk of serious complications. Related to this, how well you stick to prehab and other recommendations can make a huge difference in qualifying for transplant. It's important to dig deep and find your resolve. If you're not able to follow a basic walking and nutritional program, for instance, the likelihood of receiving an organ is lower because the surgical risks may be too great.

Whether or not a person qualifies for transplant surgery depends in part on the likelihood of complications during surgery and ability to manage postoperative recovery. Your prehab efforts will make it more likely that you qualify, but they also increase your chances of *thriving* afterward. There are plenty of survivors in the community who you may never realize received a transplanted organ. It wasn't until several years into a friendship before a coworker casually mentioned to me he'd received a transplant because of his "lousy heart."

Setting yourself up for success starts with doing your absolute best during prehab. Treat this process like your life depends on it because it essentially may. Consider this period to be the start of a life-changing—lifesaving—procedure. This is the time to find your social support group and your core, deep, intrinsic motivation.

Involve palliative care early in the process for better results. Some might see this as giving up, but that is far from the intention. It goes back to the concept of support and not going through such a stressful and anxiety-ridden time alone. Think of palliative care as nothing more than a professional support group with experience and treatments to endure this long journey. With that in mind, more than one transplant may be required. This is never what we hope for, but in certain situations, it's the reality of organ transplantation. A supportive network and positive mindset can make enough difference to matter.

DELAY SURGERY REQUIREMENT

There are unique situations where an organ match happens quickly, but for most patients this process involves some waiting, even potentially years. Each specific organ failure comes with methods for stretching out survival before a transplant procedure.

For heart failure, a left ventricular assistive device (LVAD) is a pump implanted into the heart that provides its own push for blood pressure. While implanting this device and keeping up with maintenance isn't easy, it creates a constant, even blood flow. There's a lot to keep up with, like preventing infection, monitoring fluid status, and blood volume. An LVAD isn't a fix for the core problem, to be clear, but it may buy time for qualified patients until a heart becomes available.

When facing lung failure, one aspect of management is to supplement oxygen and use a BiPAP or CPAP machine to promote better gas exchange. Liver failure involves a good amount of medication management and sometimes bypass procedures to reduce the risk of bleeding complications. When a liver isn't working correctly, the blood flowing through it causes a lot of back pressure. This causes swelling of certain blood vessels, which leads to a high risk of esophageal or rectal bleeding. Surgery is designed to bypass the problem area, but it also decreases the benefit of any remaining liver function. In other words, this is by no means a permanent fix and comes with additional medications and monitoring before transplant.

A source of hope for kidney disease and renal failure is that dialysis is improving all the time. Dialysis technology is quickly reaching a point where home-based dialysis or continuous wearable portable dialysis machines that can function like wearable kidneys are easier and available for most. Picture this future with portable dialysis machines that connect wirelessly to a kidney doctor who monitors the process and corrects electrolyte balances in real time. But even though dialysis can come to the patient and offers a temporary fix for a lot of kidney issues presently, it's still taxing on the body. Like our other methods, dialysis is not a permanent solution and simply buys time before transplant.

Pancreatic solutions involve replacing the pancreas's functions, including managing insulin and releasing digestion hormones. While we have continuous glucose monitoring and implantable insulin pumps, these aren't reliable enough to function like *true* pancreas replacements.

If you happen to be on a transplant list, there are things that can be done to maintain your health and make sure you can qualify for a new organ. However, just about all of these are temporary measures. Unless bioengineers have finally invented artificial organs, you'll still benefit from a transplant.

COMMON AND POTENTIAL COMPLICATIONS

There are more than a few complications to anticipate while preparing for an organ transplant. Neuropathy, transaminitis (high levels of liver enzymes that indicate liver injury), and cardiomyopathy (heart muscle disease) are complications that can develop after surgery and from certain medications. Antirejection medications can cause other organ injury. Some can "irritate" the kidneys, affect electrolyte levels, or raise liver enzymes (transaminitis).

This concept is kind of like how chemotherapy attacks cancer cells but also harms healthy cells in the process. These drugs can cause nerve damage that leads to pain or weakness. Your symptoms may be present going into surgery, or they could start afterward because of the treatment. This is another great reason to do your best in prehab and work with a professional who proactively addresses issues like preexisting pain, since controlling pain before surgery makes it less likely to worsen during or after treatment, or at least helps you identify medications that work for you.

Poor appetite is another byproduct of transplant surgery. This and chronic risk of illnesses are common side effects of many immunosuppressants. Immunosuppressants can also cause electrolyte wasting, tremors, infection, and potentially even higher risk for cancer down the road.

Unfortunately, transplanted organs have a life expectancy. Older organs have accumulated more damage over time, so an attempt is made to match the organ's age with the patient's age. This goes for size as well—child organs are usually smaller than adult organs.

A transplanted organ can also develop physiological changes. For example, a patient's transplanted heart may have an elevated resting heart rate and an impaired ability to increase its rate with exercise ("chronotropic incompetence"). After kidney transplant, dialysis is still required until kidney function recovers, but it will never be as good as two natural kidneys. Expect this across the board with any organ transplant—function will improve, but it won't be the same as a healthy, original organ.

Close monitoring is often required after transplant surgery. For some, there will be exercise restrictions before and after the procedure. Weight-bearing restrictions might apply, especially if we're dealing with heart or lung transplant. These are some of the most important things to prepare for. Life won't go back to "normal" but will assume a new normal that can be fulfilling with proper guidance and preparation.

There is an additional source of hope when it comes to organ transplantation. As the science behind transplants improves, the process for matching organs to patients becomes more nuanced and complex. This leads to better matches and less risk of rejection.

Ultimately, the end game is to develop artificial organs. While that may sound closer to science fiction, this isn't quite the case any longer. Some experts expect that this may come about in the next twenty or thirty years or so. Some organs are likely easier to reproduce artificially than others, allowing us to mimic their functions without relying on human donors. As of this writing, for instance, we essentially have the pieces for an artificial pancreas, as alluded to earlier; people with type 1 diabetes could potentially have a real solution in the not-so-distant future. The heart, for example, is a fairly mechanical organ. It isn't outside the realm of possibility to believe artificial hearts might exist in the next few decades. Livers perform a dizzying array of complex functions, but these may be reproducible with a mix of an artificial device and oral medications.

Exciting possibilities are on the horizon, and this domain of medicine is subject to frequent updates in the coming years as more breakthroughs occur. Prehabilitation has an important place in organ transplant for the foreseeable future, playing a role in helping patients qualify for organs and aiding them in the recovery process. One of the base principles of prehab—improving health as a way to improve quality of life—can serve patients awaiting transplant well during this process and bring them tremendous benefit.

ACTION POINTS

- Transplantation is often a long, demanding process. Once you're on a wait list for a new organ, expect finding a match to take between several weeks and a few years. This period is an opportune time to start a prehab program to improve your chances of qualifying for an organ and achieving a successful outcome.
- Depending on which organ is experiencing chronic disease or failure, there are various methods to improve quality of life and help a person live long enough to receive the transplant. Almost all of these are temporary measures that don't treat or undo the root cause of organ failure.
- Even with the best outcome possible, life after an organ transplant won't be the same as it was prior. Immunosuppressants are required for the rest of your life to prevent rejection of the new organ. While the dosage can be dialed back after recovery, these can increase the likelihood of infections and illnesses that the body has trouble fighting off. Medications can cause issues like neuropathy and harm the body's other organs. Finally, a transplanted organ offers improved function over a failing or chronically diseased organ, but it may never function the same as an original, healthy organ. This difference may not be noticeable for some.
- Science and technology are progressing toward better matching abilities with less chances of rejection and eventually producing completely artificial organs with no chance of rejection. We aren't there *yet*, but some of the required technology already exists or is well within reach.

CHAPTER 8

FERTILITY, GYNECOLOGIC SURGERY, AND UROLOGIC SURGERY PREHABILITATION

WHO THINKS ABOUT STARTING A "PREHABILITATION" PROGRAM before they get pregnant? Pregnancy is often something we take for granted. After all, well over three million Americans get pregnant each year, and more people are participating in what essentially is prehab than they likely realize.

Now, consider something like prenatal vitamins. A pregnant person doesn't start taking prenatals a day before their baby is due, nor should they even start the day they realize they're pregnant. Supplements require time to build up to appropriate levels in the bodily system to have a positive impact, and obviously, they need to be taken *prior* to creating a baby. The best times to begin prenatal vitamins are when you start trying to conceive—to build up the body's levels of key nutrients—or as soon as you find out you're pregnant. After all, preparation is key.

Prehabilitation for pregnancy works the same way. This process should start for *both* would-be parents the moment you and your partner anticipate getting pregnant. The following chapter serves to educate on how prehabilitation strategies impact pregnancy, fertility, and gynecological or pelvic surgeries. Each section is broken into two parts, the first dealing with gynecologic and pelvic surgeries, and the second dealing with fertility and obstetrics.

Gynecologic and pelvic surgeries not involving cancer typically fall under the umbrella of elective surgery. The main goal of these surgeries is to improve quality of life, which happens to be one of prehab's major objectives. Completing prehab during the preparation period improves quality of life on its own while enhancing surgery's benefits later. In other words, taking the process seriously beforehand makes living with gynecologic and pelvic issues more tolerable while awaiting surgery. It also lowers surgery risk and leads to long-term wellness. While this sometimes means delaying the ultimate relief of surgery, you'll likely feel better in the short term anyway.

On the fertility side of things, as the average individual's metabolic health worsens, rates of infertility increase. The causes stem from many factors, but a large part of this is due to hormonal changes during worsening obesity. Metabolism and hormonal signaling are very interconnected. When metabolic conditions worsen, they contribute to impaired fertility. Reversing that downward spiral is our goal, and prehab is one *seriously* effective strategy.

When it comes to fertility and pelvic floor surgery, there are more benefits to controlling metabolic disease than may meet the eye. Lowering metabolic disease means a pregnant individual is less likely to have a large baby, which will likely reduce risk of pelvic floor issues in the future. In other words, controlling metabolic disease can help avoid having a baby that's too large, which reduces the propensity for pelvic floor issues post-birth.

TREATMENT TEAM AND HELPFUL TERMINOLOGY

When preparing for gynecologic or pelvic surgery, expect to work closely with several different medical professionals. A gynecologist or urologist oversees surgery preoperative consultations and performs the actual surgery. It's good to note that some of these surgeries are minimally invasive. Much like other procedures in this book, a physical therapist (or physiatrist, if needed) will guide patients through physical preparation for surgery and recovery. This professional is often a pelvic floor rehab specialist. A nutritionist or dietician monitors a patient's nutrient intake to make sure they're making the best decisions possible for surgery and recovery. And, when needed, an endocrinologist manages the metabolic and hormonal aspects of surgery and the recovery process.

Fertility and obstetrics have a different treatment team. This is primarily made up of an obstetrician—a physician specializing in treatment of the uterus, vagina, and reproductive system—who may be a subspecialist in maternal fetal medicine (MFM) for high-risk cases or reproductive endocrinology and infertility (REI) for hormonal and procedural treatments of impaired fertility. Although not always automatically involved, a physical therapist, dietician, and exercise physiologist may incorporate crucial nutritional and physical activity-related recommendations to improve fertility and odds of achieving a healthy pregnancy. These professionals specialize in dealing with pregnancy and the recovery process, as well as exercise and weight loss to improve fertility.

Gynecologic surgery applies to any procedure related to the female reproductive system. These procedures can involve resecting (removing) fibroids, removing the uterus (hysterectomy), or treating infertility, incontinence, or several other conditions. Pelvic floor surgery is a broad term used for any procedure designed to repair the pelvic floor. The pelvic floor is a group of muscles and connective tissues attached to the bottom of the pelvic bones. It supports the organs sitting inside the pelvis. The most common dysfunction with this is pelvic organ prolapse, or when organs slip down from their normal position and impact the function of other elements of the pelvic floor. This may present as difficulty urinating, constipation, or a heaviness or achy sensation low in the pelvis.

CARE OVERVIEW

When it comes to fertility prehabilitation, the initial continuum of care starts with preconception counseling and related treatments like hormonal therapies, as needed. This leads into a relationship with your obstetrics and fertility team, who, among other roles, are responsible for dutiful monitoring throughout the preconception-pregnancy-delivery continuum. Of course, this entails a general ob-gyn but quickly extends into a number of potential subspecialists on the obstetrics side, as well as potentially a urologist for the male fertility side of things.

The female fertility side of the equation might require a professional who specializes in REI—reproductive, endocrinology, and infertility. To put it simply, these specialists work with people who have trouble getting pregnant. Their role includes different levels of counseling as well as influencing ovulatory hormone levels. They can tell if an issue arises with improper sequences of hormone fluctuations—both in the brain and body—and prescribe different medications to correct any such issues and induce ovulation when that's the issue or to troubleshoot other factors affecting fertility.

Often, metabolic disease or polycystic ovarian syndrome (PCOS) can be the underlying causes behind infertility. An REI specialist might prescribe medications to manage diabetes, for example, which will help the person lose weight and improve fertility from the metabolic side. Most of what these specialists do applies to biological females, although they are involved in artificial insemination.

On the biologically male side, a subspecialized urologist treats male infertility. Similarly, these professionals measure the hormones affecting testosterone regulation and sperm production. Their end objective is to restore normal hormonal levels so the testes produce higher quality sperm. From there, the urologist either harvests those for artificial insemination or recommends trialing "traditional" conception if sperm quality is fully recovered.

If an individual began this process as "high risk," they will still likely have other high-risk aspects of the pregnancy. Often an MFM-specialized obstetrician will continue to manage the pregnancy, as this professional focuses on high-risk pregnancies, performs risk calculations to provide prognosis estimates, and mitigates risk factors for pregnancy complications. MFMs don't just cover metabolic disease. If you're past a certain age where your age alone increases the risk of complications or you have a complication like preeclampsia or high blood pressure, you may be referred to an MFM for closer monitoring.

On the male side, once you've conceived, ongoing specialist oversight is not typically necessary, and you're free to support your partner. Research *does* suggest that exercise and good dietary practices are easier to maintain for your partner if you are continuing them yourself.[157] Just because your conception "job is done" doesn't mean your job is actually done. You're part of a team, and by helping and setting a good example, you make things easier for your partner.

As we near the due date, conversations may take place regarding inducing labor, performing a cesarean section, or having a specialized team present for delivery. These allow more control over the variables that are, obviously, often outside of our control. These scenarios quickly become very specific based on the situation. For example, if a pregnant person is older than normal but everything else is fine, a specialized team probably isn't needed. However, if someone is, for instance, carrying multiples due to IVF and delivers early, they might require a neonatologist or someone who specializes in newborns and related issues to take the newborn to the NICU (neonatal intensive care unit) for monitoring and necessary treatments.

The safety net becomes wider when there are more potential risks involved. In cases with metabolic disease, a pregnant individual is at risk for a number of known complications. These include having a large baby ("large for gestational age") that makes delivery more difficult. Early rupture of membranes can also be a cause for concern. Essentially, your water breaks too early, and this can lead to early delivery or possible loss of a pregnancy. It's important to know what has the potential to go wrong and what to expect each step of the way.

---

157 Rouhallah Rafeie et al., "Effect of Couple Education on Spouses' Anxiety and Treatment Adherence in Patients with Acute Coronary Syndrome Admitted to Cardiac Intensive Care Unit," *Medical-Surgical Nursing Journal* 10, no. 4 (2022): 1, e123617, https://doi.org/10.5812/msnj.123617; Cindy L. Carmack et al., "Healthy Moves to Improve Lifestyle Behaviors of Cancer Survivors and Their Spouses: Feasibility and Preliminary Results of Intervention Efficacy," *Nutrients* 13, no. 12 (2021): 4460, https://doi.org/10.3390/nu13124460.

Pelvic floor physical therapy may factor into the continuum of care after delivery for some individuals. This entails work with a physical therapist to rehabilitate the pelvic floor musculature by regaining strength and control. A gynecologist may come back into play and recommend treatments if there's an incontinence issue, for example. Pelvic floor dysfunction can cause incontinence, and there are several treatments to rectify this.

The care overview for pelvic surgery can vary widely because specific treatments depend on the condition that led to the surgery. For both men and women, there are many reasons to have pelvic surgery. Care begins with an obstetrician or urology consultation for whatever issue potentially requires surgery. A few of the most common are uterine fibroids; endometriosis; cancers such as uterine, prostate, and ovarian (although we go into more detail about cancer prehab in Chapter 4); and organ prolapse.

In some cases, years after delivery, the pelvic organs no longer remain suspended in their correct locations and drop lower than they should within the pelvis. This can happen to the uterus or the bladder, where it falls out of position, blocks outflow, and leads to incontinence/urinary retention. Any of these issues necessitates working with a gynecological or urogynecological surgeon, colorectal surgeon, or gynecological oncologist, in some cases. The latter are *sometimes* involved in non-cancer surgeries because they are typically experienced with performing high-risk procedures that might involve bleeding or uncertain findings. If you haven't had any conversations regarding suspected cancer, it's important to stress that having a gyn-onc surgeon present in the operation doesn't necessarily mean cancer is at play. This may be a precautionary measure or a means to involve a surgeon with a very specialized skill set that can pay dividends in these situations.

The male pelvic surgery team is led by a urologist and often deals with prostate or testicular cancer, bladder surgeries, or an enlarged prostate that requires surgery. The latter is generally no longer a traditional operation. Instead, the prostate may be treated via a transurethral resection of the prostate (TURP). Essentially, a surgeon goes through the urethra and bores out a section of the prostate to make urination easier. This type of procedure can lead to better outcomes than a full-on lower abdominal surgery, primarily because it's less invasive.

Postsurgical care, including physical therapy, is highly case dependent. Some male urologic surgeries like the TURP are generally outpatient procedures unless the patient has also had co-occurring medical decline. For example, a patient in need of a TURP because they've had frequent severe urinary tract infections may require more than a relatively simple outpatient procedure. For a patient like this, the TURP itself isn't the issue. It's simply the end of the process and leads into a rehab regimen.

In general, many urologic surgeries don't require physical therapy after surgery. However, any surgery involving the pelvic floor is likely going to come with a physical therapy component—usually outpatient—for generalized strengthening and balance, or one that's focused on the pelvic floor muscles.

PREHABILITATION PILLARS: FERTILITY AND PELVIC SURGERY

Prehab is all about doing as much as possible before a procedure or, in this case, pregnancy. This isn't only to lower the risk of complications and improve potential quality of life after surgery, but it also helps an individual feel better while preparing and allows them to work hardest before adding the strain of pregnancy or surgical recovery. Good prehab is designed to make the current situation more tolerable. This may even mean delaying the permanent relief that comes from surgery while starting to feel better in the short term. Quality of life shouldn't have to wait until after an intervention and recovery period. Some good preparation can go a long way and provide early benefit.

EXERCISE

Beyond exercising with the standard prehab goal of adding muscle and burning fat, the exercise pillar focuses on strengthening the pelvic floor within the abdominal area for pelvic stability. These muscles connect both sides of the pelvis to the urethra (the "tube" that empties the bladder) and everything inside the pelvic "bowl." These connecting muscles, ligaments, and organs create a floor that everything else sits on top of. Exercise is geared toward optimizing this stability to maintain or improve urinary continence and to prevent organs from prolapsing (falling) through this muscular floor. This is fairly common in older women who've had multiple pregnancies or delivered larger babies and may be preventable with specific pelvic floor exercises.

Resistance and aerobic training make up the bulk of the exercise pillar in a good prehab program for both pelvic surgery and pregnancy. In the latter, these are primarily used to improve the body's response to insulin, particularly in women. Exercise directly improves insulin sensitivity, and increased muscle mass gives the body more room to store sugar, indirectly reversing insulin resistance over time. However, pregnant patients with preeclampsia should not take part in resistance training without close oversight from their obstetrician so as to not run the risk of increasing blood pressure.

Some treatments require a medically induced drop in sex hormones—for individuals born biologically female, ovary removal or medications are common after certain cancers to suppress estrogen signaling, or in men a drop in testosterone when treating certain prostate cancers. These hormonal changes risk the creation of accelerated menopause or "andropause." Individuals in these situations are often faced with a risk of lower bone density, rapid loss of muscle mass, and worsening metabolic disease. Individuals in these situations must be proactive about resistance training and other weight-bearing activities to maintain bone density.

LIFESTYLE

Obesity puts added pressure on the pelvic floor muscles. Any extra abdominal weight is going to stress this part of the body and make it more difficult to "keep everything in place." Meaning one of the best strategies in this pillar is a nutritional or medicinal plan for losing weight.

Weight loss directly leads to improved continence and a host of other benefits. Sexual function for men dealing with metabolic disease tends to improve after weight loss for several reasons. One is that sexual function depends on blood flow. Smoking, diabetes, and high blood pressure can damage blood vessels and lead to decreased erectile function. Another cause is hormonal. The more fat tissue a person has, the more they convert testosterone to estrogen. In women, this raises the risk of hormone-sensitive cancers like breast and endometrial cancer. In men, it can contribute to low testosterone, low libido, poor exercise recovery, and lower energy levels, among other things.[158]

---

[158] Kristy A. Brown and Philipp E. Scherer, "Update on Adipose Tissue and Cancer," *Endocrine Reviews* 44, no. 6 (December 2023): 961–974, https://doi.org/10.1210/endrev/bnad015; Danila Coradini and Saro Oriana, "Impact of Sex Hormones Dysregulation and Adiposity on the Outcome of Postmenopausal Breast Cancer Patients," *Clinical Obesity* 11, no. 1 (February 2021): e12423, https://doi.org/10.1111/cob.12423.

For fertility and pregnancy, diabetes remains a major concern, as it has been throughout this book. A regimen focused on reversing prediabetes or diabetes should be a priority before and during pregnancy. Preconception focus should be placed on a diet rich in protein and omega fatty acids for muscle and brain development. Specific dietary recommendations during pregnancy are beyond the scope of this book and may vary based on personal circumstances. However, a high-protein diet without undercooked meat or high-mercury fish (tuna, shark, and swordfish) but including vegetables and fruits like berries and apples is a great starting point. This is important pre- and postpartum.

NEUROPSYCHIATRIC

Gynecologic and pelvic floor issues are frequent causes of chronic pain in women, with depression and anxiety often following. When it comes to men, depression and anxiety are both contributors to and causes of urologic and sexual dysfunction.

Again, the human body is full of many interconnected systems, and how the neuro pillar interacts with the rest of a good prehab program is no exception. For example, low testosterone increases the risk of depression and insomnia, but poor sleep may lower testosterone levels even further, making the problem more difficult to resolve.[159] Knowing that everything is tied together helps us come up with solutions for this pillar, such as using medications to restore testosterone back up to normal

---

[159] Rita Indirli et al., "The Association of Hypogonadism with Depression and Its Treatments," *Frontiers in Endocrinology* 14 (2023): 1–14, 1198437, https://doi.org/10.3389/fendo.2023.1198437; Adithya Balasubramanian et al., "Increased Risk of Hypogonadal Symptoms in Shift Workers with Shift Work Sleep Disorder," *Urology* 138 (April 2020): 52–59, https://doi.org/10.1016/j.urology.2019.10.040.

levels, though directly supplementing testosterone can further impair fertility. Discovering and treating the root cause is often the best, most sustainable intervention.

Some of the same issues crop up when dealing with pregnancy or fertility concerns. During this time, it's important to optimize sleep. Sleep helps regulate bodily systems and hormone levels, and it can significantly impact fertility. Getting enough restful sleep on a consistent schedule is an important part of fertility prehab. As previously mentioned, poor sleep raises many hormones that directly raise blood sugar and blood pressure, and chronically poor sleep is associated with impaired fertility in all individuals.

Many psychiatric and pain medications must often be weaned or switched to minimize potential risks during pregnancy. This could mean switching medications or tapering them off before pregnancy begins. Certain antidepressants and pain, sleep, and seizure/mood stabilizing meds are safer than others during pregnancy. Deciding which to continue and which to transition between is a risk-versus-benefit conversation between expecting parents and their medical teams.

This section wouldn't be complete without touching on stress management. Stress is not good for the baby or pregnancy. Finding ways to mitigate stress through activities like walking, therapy, and others can provide outsized returns compared to the resources required to perform them. For example, walking is a great low-impact way to improve health and relieves stress at the same time. Walking doesn't require a lot of effort—the only resource expended is time—but that stress relief and improved health can have a domino effect that leads to a healthier pregnancy.

As far as activity recommendations for pregnancy besides walking, the golden rule is to consult with your obstetrician before starting anything, especially during higher-risk pregnancies. Beyond that, for an otherwise healthy pregnancy, any activity that doesn't risk direct impact to the abdomen is acceptable. Deadlifts, running, and swimming are usually okay, after receiving your doctor's blessing. The beauty of fertility prehab is that if you've already been doing activities prior to pregnancy and know how they'll affect you, you can likely comfortably continue these activities when you're pregnant.

EXPECTATION MANAGEMENT

Not all gynecologic and pelvic floor surgeries are created equal. With different surgical methods come different recovery times and rehabilitation needs. This doesn't have much impact on how a person prepares for surgery, but the surgery type can lead to different expectations for the recovery time period.

Surgery in this field is typically broken into traditional open surgery and different minimally invasive surgery types. The latter are sometimes used in pelvic procedures and involve small cuts around half an inch long through which tubes are inserted into the abdomen or pelvis, guided by cameras (laparoscopy). Robotic surgeries are essentially the newest variations of laparoscopic surgeries. The da Vinci Surgical System is the most common robotic surgical system at the time of this writing and is used in abdominal and pelvic procedures like hysterectomies, hernia repairs, and prostate removals.

All things being equal, less invasive surgeries require less recovery time, but that doesn't mean *all* surgeries should be laparoscopic or robotic systems. The "best" approach depends on the procedure and realistic options for visualizing and accessing the target anatomy. The best thing a reader can take away is that surgery methods differ, but what is best for you will be determined by your team based on your unique situation. Weight loss prior to surgery, however, may increase the likelihood of a successful laparoscopic approach to surgery.[160]

Then there's a matter of medications. Fertility medications have become very popular in recent years.[161] Just like any other medications, they come with some potential mild to moderate downsides like mild to moderate hot flashes, headaches, and fatigue. Mood changes, nausea, and vomiting are other potential side effects. At the time of this writing, research into exercise for reducing side effects of hormonal fertility treatments is very limited. As exercise may improve similar symptoms associated with hormonal changes in menopause, you can reasonably try low risk interventions, such as exercise, both to improve fertility and manage medication side effects.[162]

Inpatient rehabilitation after pregnancy is unlikely unless a patient suffers significant complications. For example, during my training, I cared for two women who had COVID-19-related complications during pregnancy and who, after delivery, required inpatient rehabilitation. Short of something well out of the ordinary, don't expect admittance. Everyone's recovery is unique, but this provides a reasonable idea of what to expect during the recovery experience from pregnancy and pelvic surgery. Like other prehab scenarios, barring unexpected

---

[160] Sally Griffin et al., "Elective Surgery in Adult Patients with Excess Weight: Can Preoperative Dietary Interventions Improve Surgical Outcomes?," *Current Developments in Nutrition* 6, Supplement 1 (June 2022): 1059, https://doi.org/10.1093/cdn/nzac070.018.

[161] Emily Sadecki et al., "Fertility Trends and Comparisons in a Historical Cohort of US Women with Primary Infertility," *Reproductive Health* 19, no. 1 (2022): 1–11, 13, https://doi.org/10.1186/s12978-021-01313-6.

[162] T. Liu et al., "Effects of Exercise on Vasomotor Symptoms in Menopausal Women: A Systematic Review and Meta-Analysis," *Climacteric* 25, no. 6 (2022): 552–561, https://doi.org/10.1080/13697137.2022.2097865.

complications, most individuals will be discharged to recover at home.

DELAY SURGERY REQUIREMENT

Medical management is often the best tactic for delaying any type of pelvic surgery. NSAIDs like naproxen or ibuprofen are common choices for pelvic pain, given the influence of inflammatory hormones. Medications that mimic or alter the function of estrogen and progesterone are frequently used for specific things like premenstrual dysphoric disorder (PMDD), fibroids, and endometriosis. PMDD is a severe form of premenstrual syndrome (PMS). NSAIDs and birth control are used to help control this and other hormone-influenced conditions. In pregnancy, however, *only* acetaminophen (Tylenol) is safe to take for pain relief, unless meds like opioids are prescribed by a doctor.

COMMON AND POTENTIAL COMPLICATIONS

We'll break down complications into obesity-related issues, pelvic floor disorders, and fertility complications. Typical complications after a gynecologic or pelvic floor procedure include wound infection and pain. Ovarian torsion, where an ovary twists on its attachment (the fallopian tube) and cuts off blood flow, can occur during the preoperative period before ovary removal—oophorectomy—due to ovarian cysts, for example. These types of cysts aren't necessarily the same as the cysts involved in polycystic ovary syndrome (PCOS), though PCOS is a risk factor for enlarged cysts and torsion. Hormonal complications can occur after an oophorectomy of even one ovary.

In the fertility and obstetrics realm, a handful of complications can occur either before or during pregnancy. PCOS is the most common hormonal disorder that appears in women of reproductive age. PCOS is named after cysts that form on the ovaries and can contribute to infertility.

Preeclampsia is a potentially life-threatening complication that occurs during pregnancy/immediately after delivery and shows up in multiple ways, often as high blood pressure and headaches, visual changes, and large amounts of protein in the urine (this makes it especially "frothy" appearing). This disorder is specific to pregnancy and also has signs and symptoms in the form of swelling in the hands, feet, and legs. It's important to avoid strenuous exercise unless this condition is well controlled. Many symptoms associated with preeclampsia may occur in a normal, healthy pregnancy, so it is important to be diligent with prenatal visits and monitoring.

Transitioning from old medications before or during pregnancy could potentially worsen some psychological conditions. However, there is a chance that pregnancy could actually improve some health conditions. We should note that some medications held during pregnancy like immunosuppressants for rheumatoid arthritis or lupus can lead to flare-ups. For some, however, the relative changes in certain hormones and immune function actually *improve* certain conditions during pregnancy.

All of that said, preparation and knowing what you're up against are the two most effective ways to tackle any pelvic procedure or fertility obstacle. Just like most people wouldn't start prenatal vitamins midway through a pregnancy, it's best to prepare before getting pregnant or weeks in advance of a pelvic or gynecologic procedure. The prehabilitation period is like laying a solid foundation—physically and mentally—for everything that will come afterward. And just like any great foundation, it is built on sound principles and consistent implementation to have the highest chance of leading to the best outcomes.

ACTION POINTS

- Treating infertility is a process and doesn't respond well to overnight changes or extreme measures. Both partners should allow the appropriate time for consistent application of fertility and pregnancy prehabilitation.
- Steady, incremental efforts are best in this area. Poor health and habits are connected to infertility. This should be taken into account and corrected as much as possible with things like aerobic exercise, resistance training, dietary changes, and medications as needed. Extreme interventions like "crash diets" or very strenuous exercise, however, may temporarily impair fertility.
- There is a spectrum of gynecologic and pelvic floor procedures, some naturally more invasive than others. Generally, the more invasive a surgery, the more recovery time is needed. Robotic surgery systems are making progress on this front, but they aren't appropriate for all surgeries. Improve surgical benefits, reduce complications, and improve your quality of life before an intervention with prehabilitation that focuses on improved strength and physical activity, targeting metabolic diseases with nutritional improvements and weight loss.
- Complications can occur whether you're preparing for a procedure or going through pregnancy. The best way to limit complications is by controlling metabolic diseases like type 2 diabetes.
- Gynecologic and pelvic disorders are heavily influenced by specific hormones, including but not limited to estrogen, progesterone, and testosterone. These may also drop substantially *after* surgery, leading to early menopause or, in men, the similar condition called "andropause."

CHAPTER 9

OUR MISSION TO PUT HEALING FIRST

THE INTRODUCTION OF THIS BOOK PROMISED YOU A TOOL TO get back in the driver's seat. One of my main motivations for this book is to help you start your "second life." There are millions of people out there going through difficult, anxiety-ridden medical journeys who sometimes feel little hope of reaching a healthier, more fulfilling future, even with a life-changing procedure on the horizon. Health and fulfillment mean something different to every single person who reads this, but the core message rings true: at times, we could all use a figurative GPS to guide the way.

Picture the presurgical period as a series of winding roads leading up to a tunnel in the mountains. When you get started, you can vaguely see the tunnel up ahead, embedded in the side of a mountain, but from your seat, all you see is a forest of trees and dense fog or snow obstructing your view of the winding roads to get there. A multimodal prehab program is your GPS, snow tires, warm cup of coffee, and great audiobook playing in the speakers—may I even suggest this book? Suddenly the journey goes from treacherous to adventurous, and when all is said and done, you pass through the tunnel to see an open road and a beautiful view. That is the second life you've got ahead of you, ripe with opportunities to try something new with your fresh hip, relieved back pain, cancer remission, or highly functioning prosthetic.

Serious diseases and conditions sometimes strike when we're least prepared. No one is ever ready for a life-changing diagnosis or a long and arduous path of surgeries and treatments. There are things in this life we can't control, and that's something that isn't likely to change. But how you think—your mindset—isn't one of them. When you refuse to be a passenger and insist on driving your life's journey in spite of the complications and unknowns along the way, that's when you take the first step toward ridding yourself of that feeling of powerlessness. Ownership and a winning mentality lay the foundation of successful outcomes. Fighting back isn't necessarily easy—as this book has illustrated, prehabilitation involves hard work, commitment, and sacrifice—but I'd be lying if I said it wasn't worth it *every single time*. The end result is better quality of life before and after treatment and greater peace of mind more often than not. There is limited time when faced with an impending medical intervention, whether that's major surgery or other type of treatment. By making the most of that time, you're actively improving your chances of a successful outcome.

This book was crafted with a singular purpose: to empower you, the reader, or someone you love to reclaim control over your health and well-being. In almost every situation, from managing a chronic condition to simply striving for a better quality of life, the concept of prehabilitation offers a transformative approach. At its heart, prehabilitation is about proactive preparation—equipping yourself not just to endure but to thrive through medical challenges. It's about recognizing that amid the uncertainty and anxiety of medical journeys, as difficult as they can sometimes be, there exists a tangible road forward, illuminated by knowledge, preparation, and determination.

Every reader brings their own personal hopes, fears, and aspirations into this equation. Yet united by the shared desire for better health and vitality, you've turned to this book seeking guidance and understanding. Here, you've hopefully found not just information but a North Star to navigate the complexities of prehab and an arsenal of practical, strategic insights to bolster your physical, mental, and emotional resilience.

Prehabilitation is more than a preparatory phase; it's a philosophy—an affirmation of your agency in shaping your health outcomes. It empowers you to confront adversity head on, to embrace the transformative power of preparation, and to emerge stronger on the other side with a sense of pride.

Just like your path, the medical world never stands still. Medicine's rapid progression means that the tactics we use in prehab that can lead to better outcomes will only continue to evolve and improve. What seems like an insurmountable peak today may be traversed with much less effort in the near future, thanks to ongoing advancements in medical science and technology. It takes hard work, but you've got what it takes to dig deep, shift into a low gear, and climb the mountain empowered. Medicine is practically leaping forward, guiding us to a place where even more is possible.

In the meantime, the best advice I can offer is to give prehabilitation everything you've got and don't hold back. It may be difficult, but embrace this new challenge with unwavering determination knowing that it is for a relatively short, defined period, and the end is in sight. Let this book serve not just as a guide but as a beacon of hope and empowerment.

Keep climbing. Keep believing in the outcomes of your hard work. Your journey toward improved health and overcoming your obstacles begins now. You can do it!

ACKNOWLEDGMENTS

IN THE VEIN OF "IT TAKES A VILLAGE TO RAISE A CHILD," OVER the past few years, this book has become my child—waking me in the middle of the night in a cold sweat, starting as an amorphous blob with limitless potential and becoming something of which I couldn't be more proud.

Taking this further, I've received direct and indirect help from more people than I could adequately thank in dozens of pages. My beautiful and supportive wife, Alia, of course, deserves the most gratitude within this village for being my cheerleader, counselor, confidant, and consoler through the most challenging moments of this project. Life happens and can make priorities like this one seem trivial. Yet you not only excused my absences from swimming lessons and bedtime stories, but you also kept me going during heavier moments that would have distracted even the most focused stoics. Thank you for believing in every far-fetched dream we've shared together, my love.

The rest of my immediate and extended families, our friends, and the whole Admire Medical crew warrant substantial gratitude as well. My sister, Lauren, deserves particular mention for rallying behind this book and seeing what it could become with the necessary investment of our limited time and energy. The exciting work we've already accomplished together at Admire is nothing compared to what's coming next.

Finally, I'd like to thank everyone who contributed to the companion textbook on which this book is loosely modeled, *A Prehabilitation Guide for All Providers*. It was a privilege working with all these distinguished experts but especially my co-editor, Dr. Karen Barr. Karen, you encouraged me to turn an elective month during my final year of residency into the first comprehensive resource for this growing subspecialty. Before that, however, you were the first to connect the dots for me between self-study and the actual clinical practice of prehabilitation, inspiring my love for the hopefulness and empowerment it provides our patients.

Thank you all.

ABOUT THE AUTHOR

New Jersey native DR. ALEXANDER WATSON attended the University of Pennsylvania for premedical studies before returning home and completing a combined MD/MBA program at Rutgers, the State University of New Jersey. During his residency at the University of Pittsburgh Medical Center (UPMC), Dr. Watson was fortunate to train with leaders in the spaces of physical medicine & rehabilitation (PM&R), interventional/noninterventional pain management, obesity medicine, and prehabilitation. He used his business background to weave these medical fields into a specialty practice in Middletown, Delaware—Admire Medical.

At Admire, Dr. Watson and his team are obsessed with developing innovative ways for delivering life-transforming medical care. In addition to medical practice, Admire Medical is privileged to pay it forward through multiple books, formal lectures, and podcasts like the *Do Something Admirable Podcast* and *Building Something Admirable*. In the latter media, Dr. Watson and guests share prehabilitation/obesity medicine and business startup insights, respectively, to aid other patients and practices in finding their success within a restrictive, insurance-driven US healthcare system.

www.ingramcontent.com/pod-product-compliance
Lightning Source LLC
Chambersburg PA
CBHW051532020426
42333CB00016B/1896